Zacharias Tanee Fomum

INNER HEALING

Éditions du Livre Chrétien
4, rue du Révérend Père Cloarec
92400 Courbevoie France
editionlivrechretien@gmail.com

First Edition. 1988, 3500 Copies

Printed by :

Editions du livre chrétien

4, rue du Révérend Père Cloarec

92400 Courbevoie - FRANCE

Tél : (33) 9 52 29 27 72

Email : editionlivrechretien@gmail.com

Cover by :

Jacques Maré

I dedicate this book, with love, to

Roger Heim,

a man after God's heart,

my friend and

my wise and loving counsellor.

Table of Contents

Dedication..5
Preface..9
Part Two: Testimonies..11
Part Two: Disappointments..33
Part Three: God's answers to disappointments -1....................41
Part Four: God's answers to disappointments - 2....................49
Part Five: Guilt and inner healing....................................57
Part Six : The sins of parents and inner healing....................69
Part Seven: Forgiving others and inner healing....................77
Part Eight: The Impact of childhood on adult life....................83
Part Nine: God's provision for the problems of childhood.......91
Part Ten: Rejection in adult life and healing from it.............99
Part Eleven: Comparison and its consequences....................107
Part Twelve: Inner health in perpetuity....................................121

Preface

There are many people who are physically sick. Some have diseases that are visible from the outside of their bodies while others have diseases that are hidden inside their bodies. These need healing. Jesus Christ is the Answer to their need.

There are other people whose sicknesses are deeper than the physical dimension. They are crippled by fear, bitterness, jealousy and the like. Psychologists are doing the best that they can to provide answers for these people.

We, however, believe that Jesus is the right Answer for these people as well. He is God's Answer to all of man's need of healing and health. He has provided in His death, resurrection and enthronement, all that man needs for total healing at all levels.

The believer is called to enter into all that the Lord Jesus has provided for his total healing. He must co-operate with the Lord Jesus in order to enter into all that the Lord has provided for him. Sometimes this co-operation will demand that he, too, like his Lord, take up his cross, follow his Lord and die on it - to his love of "self" in all its forms. Out of this death comes, not only perfect inner healing, but also perfect inner health in perpetuity.

This book is a modest attempt to enable the believer to receive inner healing and enjoy inner health.

I consider it a great privilege to have been used by the Lord to minister to His children through this book. It is my prayer that it should help some who are bound by fear, jealousy, bitterness, lovelessness and the like, to enter into the glorious liberty of the sons of God.

Yaounde,
13th September 1986.

Dr Zacharias Tanee Fomum
B. P 6090
Yaoundé – Cameroun

PART ONE

Testimonies

1. FIRST TESTIMONY

My mother was engaged to be married to a certain young man of her choice. Shortly after their engagement, this young man's father, who was a friend to my grandfather, came to see him to say that he himself wanted to marry my mother, his reason being that women grow old faster than men and that no sooner would they be married than my mother would appear older than his son. Without consulting my mother, my grandfather agreed with his friend and a date was fixed for my mother to be taken to him as the ninth wife. When the news got to my mother, she cried and begged and did all that was in her power, but my grandfather was the kind of man whose word was law law. None of his wives could change or influence any of his decisions. They all feared him. My grandmother was afraid to oppose the idea, so she begged my mother to accept in order to spare the lives of both of them. Finally, to satisfy her parents, (though she had no choice) my mother consented to this arrangement and on the appointed day she was taken to her "father husband", who was about my grandfather's age or even older. He had children who were older than my mother and his first eight wives were far older than her, others even older than my grandmother.

About two years after she got married, my mother found that she could not bear the life she led in that home. So she ran back to her parents. All attempts to get her back to her husband failed, so she stayed with her parents. It was at this time that she met my father. They had not gone out for long when she got pregnant. When she told my father about the pregnancy, he took the news very badly and with a lot of anger. If I remember very well, he even suggested that my mother get rid of the baby (that is, me). When my mother refused, he sent her away very cruelly and asked her never to set foot in his house again. This ended their short-lived relationship. Some months later, when my mother was quite heavy with her pregnancy, my father's new girlfriend and her friends caught my mother and got her well beaten. On another occasion, my mother went to a shop to buy the last things that she needed for her baby who was due in a few days. When she went into the shop, my father was there. When he saw her, he walked out without a word. That was the last day they saw each other until 15 years later.

When my father backed out of my mother's life, there was another man who had been very interested in her but my grandmother had never wanted to see him. This was before my mother's marriage. When this man heard all that my mother was going through, he made his appearance again and decided to shoulder the responsibility. So he came many times to see her, bringing presents almost every time he came. His relatives knew my mother very well and believed that the baby was theirs. When I was finally born, he came, this time not only with presents but with a name for me. The name he gave me, when interpreted, meant that I had come as a comforter to my mother. I bore this name for two weeks.

When my mother's former husband heard that my mother had had a baby, he made haste to come with a name, saying that, according to tradition, since he had paid a brideprice for my mother, all the children my mother would ever have would belong to him, unless his money was reimbursed and, of course, he refused all reimbursements, because he had his plans to kill my mother, my elder brother (his son) and me through sorcery. So he refused to take back his money as this would take away all the claims he had over us. Then he came along with his own names. My grandfather immediately gave in and my names were changed. I was going to be called from that time on .... I bore these names until I reached school age and had to go to school. My grandmother had not been in agreement with the fact that this man had given me names, so she secretly arranged with her relative who was the headmaster of the school I was to attend and he removed the man's names and gave me new names. I was now known as.......

When I passed to class 3 (primary school) my mother, who was now married to her second husband, was moving to another part of the country with her husband. She could not take me along because it was mid-academic year and, secondly, she was not sure of the school facilities in her new locality. She left me with her sister so that I could finish that academic year. At this point, I had to be moved from my old school to join my aunt's children in the school they attended. My aunt's daughter (she was my age) and I decided to change my names so that I should bear her father's name because, according to us, we had become sisters. Fortunately, my aunt stepped in on time to stop this crazy venture.

When I finally moved to meet my mother, I was registered in school with a new name. I now bore my step-father's name. Once more my names changed, now to ...... I bore this name until I got to Form four in secondary school when my maternal uncles insisted that the names be changed so that this man's name should not appear on my G.C.E certificate. An age declaration was made then by my uncles and my grandfather's name was given as my father's name. From then on, I bore my grandfather's name. I was now .... until I got married and finally changed names for the last time.

Now, it happened that when I went to college my father's relative was in the same college. Very often this relative remarked that I very much resembled her relative. Time and again, she would jokingly say, "I am afraid there is a mistake somewhere. This kind of resemblance cannot be a mere coincidence." To me, it didn't mean anything. After all, many people thought that I also looked very much, in fact, exactly like my maternal grandmother. Anyway, when I came home for holidays, I told my mother about this girl and how she kept repeating the fact that I resembled her relative. In telling her, I attached no importance to it. It was just a conversation, but I noticed that my mother, after inquiring about the girl's tribe and family, got very vexed and said, "Let her stop it, let them not eat you through their sorcery." On my part, I attached no strings to my mother's vexation. Life went on and everything was forgotten till holidays were over and I went back to school.

When I went back to school, that girl and I got friendlier with each other. One day we went out and, by chance, we met this relative of hers. She stopped him and when we went across the road and greeted him, she said, "Here is the girl I have always talked to you about. Don't you think she resembles you?" His friend who was with him agreed very strongly and expressed his surprise at such a "coincidence". This man on his part physically trembled. He asked me many questions like: Who my mother was, where she was at the time, what she was doing, when I was born, etc. Well, I answered all of these questions without any reservations. There was no fear or suspicion in my heart.

During the holidays, I once again told my mother about this strange meeting with this man. Again, my mother was very angry, but it meant very little to me. But, one day, during that holiday, just after my mother had gone to work and I was cleaning outside the house, this man arrived. At that time, I had very many suitors and the whole thing about marriage didn't appeal to me at all. In fact, it annoyed me. So, when I saw this man, I feared that he had also come to file in his candidature. At that thought, I stiffened up and became very nervous. Anyway, I had to force through some politeness. I had been brought up and taught never to be impolite to anybody. I was very surprised that he knew our house, and I wondered how he had found his way there. I greeted him and showed him in. After a short while, he asked about my mother, and I told him that she had gone to work. He asked if I could take him to her job site and I agreed and we left. In the car, he asked me whether I knew my father. I told him I did. He asked me where my supposed father was, and I told him. He asked me who had shown me my father. At that point my patience and courtesy were beginning to run out. I almost rudely said I had known my father right from childhood, that my mother had shown him to me, and that I knew him and he knew me. At this point our interview stopped until we reached our destination.

As soon as the car stopped, I jumped out and rushed into the building and asked for my mother. When she arrived, I said, almost out of breath, "Mama, you remember that man I told you about?" She asked, "Which man?" "The one I said his relative at school thought I resembled," I replied. "And what about him?" my mother asked. I replied, "He is here. He is outside. He came to the house and asked if I could bring him to you." On hearing these words my mother's countenance dropped. However, we both came out. They both greeted each other like old acquaintances and walked a few metres away to talk. Even then, that meant very little to me. After all, my mother knew many people. He could be one of her old acquaintances. They talked for a few minutes and the man took me back home.

On our way back, he was the first to speak. All the while I was hoping that he wasn't a suitor. When he broke the silence, he said, "You can see that your mother and I have known ourselves before, can't you?" I answered, "Well, from the way you greeted yourselves it is evident that you are old friends." He took the opportunity to inform me that they knew themselves before I was born. This brought some relief to me because I thought that if he knew my mother before I was born, he couldn't be coming to ask for my hand in marriage. I was surprised that he looked so young.

That very day, he came back in the evening to talk with my mother. They went outside the house where they argued for hours.

This went on daily for one week. My fears returned and became intensified. Maybe he really wanted to marry me. After all, there were men who looked for very little girls to marry. I really feared that this could be the case. On the last day of that week, he came to tell me that he was going to the town from where he had come, but that he was coming back in two weeks.

After two weeks, he came back. This time, he came determined to make himself known to me. He resumed his daily visits and arguments with my mother. One evening, he came with six bottles of assorted whiskies. This intensified my fears. My mother kept the drinks in the cupboard, but said nothing to me. She wanted to consult her brother about whether or not to introduce my father to me. When she told her brother, he gave a furious "No" and even threatened to do harm if by any chance he met my father in our house. So my mother told my father that she was sorry she wasn't going to let me know anything about him being my father. My father didn't take it nicely. He decided to take the issue of introducing himself into his hands. So he kept on visiting us daily until the day of his return to his town of residence. That day he decided to come very early in the morning.

When my mother saw him, she got very angry and ordered him to get out of her house. In replying he said, "Yes, I am going out, but before I go," turning to me, he added, "Ask your mother to tell you who I am." As if she was expecting that, my mother answered before he had even finished, "He is your father, but ask him where he is coming from, where he has been all these years." Of course, a bitter quarrel broke out between them. I just sat there blank as if I had been dreaming, totally shocked and in wonder. Suddenly, I felt very strong hatred rising within me, against this father I had just discovered. He tried to mumble a few words of explanation and excuse, but this only earned him more hatred and contempt from me. I didn't say a word. After a few other exchanges of words between them they left; first my father, then my mother.

This was only the beginning of real conflicts in me. I had always loved my first father very much. It was very difficult to think that he was not really my father, and that this man whom I hated with every cell of my being was my father. I didn't want to ever see him again. From time to time he tried to visit me and give me presents, but I rejected him and all his presents in cash or kind. He tried to use other people to calm my mother and me, but these attempts proved futile.

The idea of belonging to two fathers now tore me into shreds.

The one I loved so much wasn't my true father. The one I hated bitterly was my father. Then a feeling of belonging to no one crept into my heart and created a sense of deep insecurity. This later on influenced my life very much.

I started seeking security to the extent that when I fell in love and got married, I got over-attached to my husband. I thought the feeling of insecurity in me could be taken away if my husband gave me all his attention. I desired and demanded so much love and attention from my husband that, when I thought that I was not having as much as I needed or desired, I would withdraw into myself for days, feeling very frustrated and sick. I was looking for a father in my husband, in addition to a lover. Of course, my husband could never be my father. I was greatly in need of inner healing - healing from the wounds caused by the shocks I had had which had created some insatiable emotional vacuum in me. I wanted my husband all to myself and didn't want anyone or anything else to have any bit of his attention. This only opened me up for more shocks and wounds, because it wasn't possible that my husband give all his attention to me alone.

I got so terribly embarrassed as I thought of how many times my names had been changed. I looked at my birth certificate and in the place of my father's name, it was my grandfather's name. A feeling of belonging to no one and to nowhere seized my heart. I didn't see my place in the society any more. I became dissatisfied and bitter. I was really hurt inside. I no longer felt comfortable in the company of friends when they talked about their fathers. I felt even worse each time I was asked my name. The idea of my grandfather's name as my father's name embarrassed and revolted me. I was bleeding inside.

But thanks be to God, in the midst of this inward battle, I met Jesus as my Lord and Saviour. I got reconciled to God through Him. As I continued with the Lord and in fellowship with other believers, I got to learn that God was not interested in taking only my sins away, but that He is interested in everything concerning me. God wanted me to cast all my frustrations, all my embarrassments, all my shame and all that kept me uncomfortable, on Him. I found a more mature believer and opened my heart's bitterness to her. Together, we lifted up to God one shock after the other. We told God about all that embarrassed me and caused me shame. This took us a number of meetings together to talk and to pray. God, in His faithfulness, heard us, and took away all the bitterness and hurt and made me see that I could never have been an accident because in His creation there are no accidents. I was in God's plan in His creation. It wasn't an accident when my mother met my father. God, who is all-knowing, knew that out of that relationship, one of His creatures would come. When God opened my eyes to see that, my pains departed. I got healed from inner hurts and the frustration departed. God also granted me the grace to forgive my father, and also brought me to begin to love him and to accept myself, not as some unwanted child, but as one who is wonderfully and fearfully made by God. Now I talk about these things, not with embarrassment, but with the joy of having known God's healing touch, and the joy that my life is a manifestation of God's sovereignty. Left to my mother, my father was never going to know me, but God, in His sovereignty, arranged for me to resemble my father. He arranged the first and the subsequent meetings with him. Above all, in His sovereign power, He healed me of all my hurts, shocks, frustrations and embarrassments. He delivered me from bitterness and hatred and from an unforgiving spirit (heart) and filled my heart with love and a capacity to forgive.

Glory be to Him!

2. SECOND TESTIMONY

Through this testimony, I would like to tell of how much God has been good to me. I have come to know God as the God of love, mercy and grace. He has forgiven my sins and has taken away my guilt. He has also healed me of my inner hurts. Today, when I look back, I am amazed at all that God has done for me.

When I received the Lord, I realized that there were certain abnormal things in my life. I was proud and very secretive. I did not like that other people should know my failures. I liked giving the impression that all was fine. Consequently, I was a liar and a hypocrite. It was only much later that I understood the origin of my problem.

I had withdrawn into myself due to the atmosphere that reigned in my parents' home. The memory I have of my childhood is that of an unhappy home, where my father and mother often fought. My father was often absent from home due to his job. When he came home, there was nagging and fighting. My mother cried very often. Each time my father had a new girl-friend, he usually abandoned home to live with her. He would only come home to spend a few nights or to bring his dirty clothes for my mother to wash. This situation terribly weighed on me. I loved my father very much and he also loved me, but sometimes I wished that he would die so that we would have peace at home.

Whenever my parents started fighting, all the children would start crying. Sometimes I gave him little punches on the back because I didn't know what else I could do. Sometimes I told my mother to leave home. In the house I was sorrowful and silent, but at school I was quite a different person. I laughed with my friends and was very talkative. I talked about everything with my classmates, but I never said a word about my family. I was very ashamed of my family. I carefully hid all that was happening at home and started loving my family as one would love a crippled child.

My elder brother, the oldest boy in the family, abandoned his studies in Form One and started stealing. He was imprisoned quite a number of times. These things made me very ashamed and I never wanted to talk about them with anybody. At one time, my elder brother, together with my two other brothers, stole from the house of the principal of the High School. All three of them almost went to prison. It was terrible. At home, my father scolded all the time, and always beat my brothers. Sometimes, he took them himself to the Police Post to have them beaten. At home, all the children talked very little. Only my younger brother expressed himself freely. Each one of us lived his or her own life. Although there was affection in our hearts for each other, we never expressed those feelings. Some kind of unexpressed modesty kept us from exposing our feelings. Our parents never expressed their feelings either. So I grew up, considering love a shameful and despicable feeling. To me, one could love but should not admit it. Unconsciously, I was likening love to weakness. I despised those girls who went out with boys under the pretext that they were in love. I was surprised to find girls in Form Four going out with Form Three boys, for example.

On the other hand, there was practically no dialogue between my father and his children. When we needed anything, we passed through our mother to tell him. In return, he talked to us through the intermediary of our mother. So I grew up without the knowledge of paternal authority; on the one hand, because my father was almost never at home and, on the other hand, because he almost never spoke to me. As far as decisions on important issues in life were concerned, I decided for myself. After Form Four, I decided that I was going to continue my studies at the Yaounde Technical High School. To this my father readily agreed.

While I was in the Lower-Sixth Form, something happened which shattered me completely. This was my elder sister's divorce. I could not understand. Was it therefore an impossibility to find a happy home around me? Was happiness in marriage just utopia?

I was bitter. I blamed all the men. I felt sorry for my sister and her three children. In my opinion, life was meaningless and suicide seemed to me the best method of ending it all. In class, my performance dropped from bad to worse. I spent a lot of time studying, but my results were mediocre, such that I failed the Advanced Level (Baccalaureate).

I started looking for something that could fill the emptiness which I felt in my heart. I needed to come out of my loneliness. I needed someone who would love and understand me. I feared men because I thought they were all alike, i.e. selfish and liars. Each time a boy approached me, I thought he had only one thing in mind - sexual intercourse. This made me very cautious. Sometimes I tried to overcome these fears, but they still came and hindered my building any relationship with the opposite sex. On the other hand, I found nothing attractive in men. Somehow, I felt that if I found a boy who truly loved me, and who could bring a solution to all my problems, then I might find life interesting. But I felt that maybe sincere and faithful men only existed in fairy tales. Sometimes, I felt such hatred for men that I told myself, "I will marry for one purpose, that of making my husband suffer and, as such, pay for all that my mother and sister have suffered."

I was lonely and unhappy. I did not even have a friend in whom I could confide my problems. Besides, I did not want to talk about them. I started visiting night clubs with one of my cousins who was in the habit of going to such places. My goal was to visit all the night clubs in town, hoping to find in them some satisfaction. I also began to think that there was something satisfying in sexual intercourse, something that could fill my emptiness. So I decided to try it. To calm my conscience, I told myself that it was one means of revenging on men. It was useless to preserve one's virginity for the sake of a man, who was not any better than the others. Having decided, I had only to choose the partner with whom to go into such an experience. It was difficult to choose because I had no affection for anybody. So, I finally chose one boy who was courting me and whom I found to be handsome. After the experience, I was more disappointed and resolved never to be involved in a sexual relationship again. It had given me no pleasure, and I even wondered what others found in it to the extent of being enslaved by it.

It was at this point of total disillusionment that a young girl talked to me about the Lord Jesus. I heard all that she said but did not understand anything. I told her that I was also a Christian and that I even had a Bible. We started having prayer meetings in the dormitory. I attended those meetings, and even prayed during the meetings, but no change had taken place in my heart. One day, this young girl invited me to an evangelistic meeting and I accepted her invitation. At the meeting, the preacher talked about the love of Jesus Christ for sinners. While he was speaking, it was as if a bright light suddenly shone within me. I understood that Jesus had died for my sins. I understood that before God, He had taken my place and suffered the punishment that I deserved because of my sins. That message was new to me. I had heard many people say that Jesus had died for us, but it had meant nothing to me. I had always known that there is a God. I very much wanted to walk in His ways, but I was unable to. I received confirmation, hoping that it would draw me nearer to God. But after my confirmation, I even became worse. Sometimes, I even said publicly that Jesus Christ was a white man and that I had nothing to do with Him. However, I feared God, having come to the knowledge of His precepts through the reading of the Old Testament. I would have liked to throw myself headlong into sin like all the other young girls I knew, but within me, there was always the fear of judgment. Hence I was torn apart between God's law (precepts) and the powerful inclination to sin which I was unable to overcome.

At the evangelistic meeting that Sunday, I understood that I did not have to put in any effort to become better. I understood that, while I was still a sinner, Christ died for me. I only had to believe it and I would be free from the power of sin. I believed it, and asked Christ to come into my life and help me to live His life. That evening, as I came out of the hall, I knew some radical change had taken place in me. When I got home, I told my elder sister that I had received Jesus Christ in my heart and that I was no longer the same. She did not understand what I was talking about, but soon after that, she realized that I had changed. I got up very early to read my Bible and pray. In the evenings, I gathered all the children and read the Word of God to them. I had become very joyful and talked about nothing but my Saviour. I was sure that from then on, I had eternal life. All my sins had been forgiven. Now, life had become meaningful. I was no longer alone. Jesus Christ and all those who loved Him were around me.

Nevertheless, I was still very proud and independent. I continued doing just whatever pleased me. Jesus Christ was my Saviour, but not my Lord. In the depth of my being, I felt no deep gratitude for the fact that I had been saved. I told myself that I had not gone as deep into sin as other girls of my age. I had only committed fornication once, and to me, this was not very serious. There was no deep humility in my heart before God. Anything that I wanted to do for the Lord, I wanted to do it for His glory and for mine too. I always wanted to exalt myself above others. I had no compassion for the weaknesses of others.

After my Advanced Levels (Baccalaureate) I decided to register for Economic Sciences at the University. This was because I despised those who studied Arts. The Lord humbled me by allowing that I "burn my mandate" after three years (i.e. failure to the point of being dismissed.)

This pride and independence, which I had cultivated from childhood, caused me to suffer a lot of pain, which God used to break me, and then heal me. It all started just before our marriage and continued after.

After our marriage, my husband and I were both frustrated and bitter. In particular, I blamed some brethren who had opposed our marriage. I was very bitter, and in my bitterness my spiritual life was at the lowest ebb. I had lost all contact with God. I justified all my actions and accused everybody for being responsible for my bad condition. I felt that no one had sought to understand me. I specially blamed those who, instead of minding their own affairs, caused disorder in others' lives by intruding. I had always thought that in life, each person had to mind his or her own business. Personally, I had little worry about knowing other people's affairs. That was my philosophy in life. Later, I learnt that this philosophy had no place in the Christian life. We are all each other's keepers.

Since I did not want that other people should know what was happening in my parents' home, I never asked them any questions. In this way, I developed total indifference towards other people's problems. When I believed in the Lord Jesus, I still maintained this indifference to things and happenings.

Right from the beginning of our marriage, we had a lot of shocks because my husband felt that I was not submissive. He was very hard on me and blamed me in everything. At times, I did not know what to do since everything I did brought discontentment. I was always humiliated and ridiculed even in the presence of other people. You can imagine what hurt it caused in someone like me who had been used to showing people only the good side of things. I started being very afraid of my husband. I lost all self-confidence. Since I realized that it was useless to be stubborn with my husband, I opted for submission and things became a bit better. I realized that the more I accepted to be humble before him, the more tender he became. But the situation was still very difficult for me. I was continually ridiculed, nagged at and humiliated. I thought that even a child could have been better treated. I had no right to my husband's confidential affairs. Whenever I asked him a question, most often he would not answer, or if he condescended to answer me, it was by asking a question in return, and in a tone that left me ice-cold. So, I decided not to ask him any questions again and always made sure that I did not speak to him in the presence of other people. I feared being humiliated and snobbed at. Consequently, I grew more and more timid. I became artificial and was always on edge. Most of the time, I was weeping. I was inhabited by fear. Whenever my husband opened the door to our bedroom when I was sleeping, I startled.

Perhaps because I knew that all the things my husband accused me of were true or perhaps because I wanted peace, I started confessing that I was all that he said I was. I started seeing that there was nothing good in me. I was sick and hurt, and my teeth were always clenched. I thought of my ruined life, of my youth which was passing away without any goal, of my dreams which may never materialize and I wept bitterly. At times, I thought of going back to my parents, but the thought of what they would say held me back, since I had told them that true happiness could only be found in Jesus.

There was no one around me in whom I could confide. I had a friend whom I loved very much, but I had scruples about going to complain to her all the time. More over, I had maintained the habit of keeping up appearances. I did not want people to know what was happening in our home. I did not want people to look on me with pity and I did not want them to speak evil of the husband whom I respected and wanted others to respect. So, I bore all these things, which were sometimes above me; bearing them partly because I knew that if I stopped supporting our home, it would be a tragedy and partly because I was afraid of what people would say.

If, at least, things were fine in my walk with the Lord, I could have hoped that something could happen. But dark clouds had covered my sky and nothing seemed to dissipate them. Night and day, I was being eaten up by the guilt of the impurity my husband and I had committed during our courtship. I had allowed him to touch and caress me during our courtship and I could not forgive myself for it. To me, that was betraying the Lord because I knew that it was wrong and had always condemned that sort of thing very strongly. I do not know how many times I confessed and re-confessed this sin to God. I also asked my husband many times to forgive me for the harm I did to him by being light. I felt that impurity had hurt our relationship in a very deep way. I felt that it partly explained why my husband was so hard towards me. I would have given all the gold in the world for the possibility that these things never happened. Alas! the harm had been done. Together, we repented of this sin and asked God to forgive us and to heal us of its consequences. My husband had also been aware of the gravity of our sin.

I also repented of all the lies and the false impressions that I had given people. I had given the impression that I did not love my husband, whereas I did. I was behaving as though I were submitting reluctantly to some evil thing that was happening to me. The truth was that I was ashamed to love. I admired many people who were liberated in this area. Before coming to the knowledge of the Lord, I had always been ashamed to be seen in the company of a man. When I became a child of God, this feeling of shame about a love affair between the opposite sexes was re-enforced. I could not understand how one could love God and yet get married and have children. I always wondered what other believers would think about me when they found me caught in the trap of love. I had passed for someone very spiritual and I thought that others also considered me as such.

God had to be very hard in dealing with me in all these areas of pride.

God pitied me and intervened in my situation. In our home, things started to improve. Then suddenly got went worse again. There was such terrible tension between my husband and me that, unable to bear them any longer, I started telling people about all that was happening. One day, it became obvious to me that there was something false in our marriage. I had also refused this idea because it was a horrible thing. The lack of peace and the agony I felt, I blamed on the devil's manoeuvres. My hypocritical behaviour, coupled with the impurity mentioned before, contributed to the lack of peace in me. I was unable to shake off the guilt of this sin. Thinking over some of the incidents that had taken place during our wedding, I realized that I had disobeyed God in getting married. This is because

I considered some of the things that happened (particularly the opposition of the brethren), as an indication that we had to wait. The realization of this fact made me very afraid, especially as in the Assembly, we got messages which exposed the dangers of being in God's permissive will. The fear of having failed God gripped me. I did not like failure, or rather, I did not like to admit that I had failed. To admit that I had made a mistake was to admit that I had failed and I did not like that. Moreover, marriage was such an important thing that a failure there was too great a failure. I did not want to face things squarely, not even when my husband told me that we were incompatible. According to him, I was disorderly, I was not spiritual, I banged doors instead of closing them, etc. All this made me sick, depressed and sad. I was in permanent agony. There was a mixed feeling of emptiness and fear in my heart. Inspite of this, I still refused to repent. It would have been easy to tell the Lord that I had realized my independence from Him. In getting married, it had been for myself not for the Lord, since I had not wanted to wait to seek His perfect will about it.

One day, during a worship service , one brother shared with the assembly from Isaiah 54. From his sharing I knew God was talking to me. Through this brother's sharing, the Lord made me understand that He knew my situation and He was calling me again to Himself. The Lord spoke to me of forgiveness, I, who deserved judgment. He spoke to me of love and restoration. I will never forget the effect that those words had in my life. I broke down in the face of God's love. He had waited for me to repent. He was taking the first step and was granting me His forgiveness. There was nothing else I could do but to humble myself before the Lord. I confessed my hypocrisy, my lies and my disobedience from the time I had known Him. I confessed my rebellion in marrying for myself and not for Him.

After confessing these sins, I felt liberated. I asked the Lord to make my husband anew and to heal our home. I was sure that God could grant us to begin afresh in Him. God revealed Himself to me as a God of mercy and grace; for not only did He forgive me, but

He healed me and healed our home. I do not know what exactly took place, but I know that a miracle took place in my life and in our home. My husband and I often talk about these things and we never cease to praise God for what He did for us. Things just radically changed.

Some time after I had confessed my sins, my husband asked that we go on a one week of fasting and prayer. In the course of that week, we spoke very frankly with each other and I understood what was at the origin of all our grievances. The enemy was opposing us and we agreed to break all his opposition in our relationship. We knew that we loved each other but there was always a barrier between us. We were unable to express our mutual sentiments. There was always some discomfort between us which worsened when there was a third person. My husband told me that when he was coming home, he was full of the desire to see me, but when he saw me, he became hard and could not even smile. On my part, I was bound at the emotional level. I could not welcome him with a smile. We were both emotionally sick. My husband had had several hurts in his life. This made him hard and proud. We prayed about all these things, asking God to heal us. That week of prayer was quite attacked by the evil one. At one time we both got so angry that we almost stopped our fast. But the Lord sustained us.

Not long after this, we were given messages on inner healing in the church. The Lord led me to talk with my husband. We talked on two occasions during which I opened my heart to him in a way that I had never done before. For the first time, I presented the true picture of myself. As I was talking, I was also discovering who I was. I had never accepted myself for who I was. I had always sought to give a different image of myself to people. My true person with all her failures was buried in the depth of my being. I had hidden myself from me as much as I had hidden myself from others. For the first time, I saw myself for who I was and accepted it. I said to the Lord, "Lord, this person whom I am describing, this person who had led this life of hypocrisy, is me. I accept myself as I am." I also accepted my family for what it was. I understood that I was nothing and only the grace of God could have made me into a child of God. I no longer saw myself better than others. I confessed all that I had done to the Lord. I confessed to Him what I was. I pleaded for forgiveness. After that, I felt light and happy. I was very grateful to the Lord for His grace.

At home, things began to improve between my husband and me. I was very happy because, after knowing all that I was, my husband did not reject me. Instead, he accepted me. In our sexual relationship there was greater harmony. Things evolved very rapidly. To me, it was a miracle. My husband changed completely. I too changed totally.

The Lord permitted us a six months' separation from each other; for I had to go to England for a language course. During this period of separation, God moved mightily in each of us. We both understood that we loved each other and the Lord opened our eyes to see how wonderful the other partner was. I also started to pray daily for our home, asking God for total healing. I also praised God for all that He had already done and I was convinced that with Him nothing was impossible. During this period, I also learnt that nothing was as fast in its effect and as powerful as prayer. I remember that once I prayed that God would reveal to my husband that besides our usual communication by phone I needed a letter from him. A few days later, my husband called to tell me that he had understood why he had to write to me. He wrote to me a number of times, even though he normally never likes writing letters. He wrote me the most wonderful declaration of love that I have ever received from him. He also opened up and made known to me all the details of his life. At last, I came to know the things that had left a mark on his life, things that had deformed his character. Now he has confidence in me and tells me all his projects. He considers me a responsible person and he is proud of me, too.

At home, the atmosphere is relaxed. We are happy and liberated.

I sing all the time. My husband, too, does the same. Our praying together draws us closer and closer to each other. I am opening up more and more. I am no longer afraid of my husband. Now I express myself, I laugh, and I even tease him. Miraculously, the Lord has lifted the discomfort that existed between us. When I make a mistake, I no longer need to lie as I did before or cover things up with well selected words. The Lord has also liberated me from an unforgiving spirit.

God alone could have done all these things. God has given me a husband in Him, a man whom I love and for whom I pray.

I will like to shout it out to the whole world that God is alive and that, today, He still performs miracles. He heals broken hearts and broken homes. He forgives rebels and blesses them. What a God! He is the God of mercy and grace! To Him be all the glory!

PART TWO

Disappointment !

Have you ever been disappointed? It could have happened in a number of ways, including the following:

1. You did not get the education you would have liked to get. You might have wanted to have a High School diploma, a University degree, a post-graduate degree, etc. However, things did not work out that way. It could be that your parents were not rich enough to pay for your education up to the level you had desired. It could be that you went to school where the conditions were poor and you were not taught by qualified teachers. This resulted in your failing to pass the University entrance examination. It could be that the educational system changed just before you entered the final year. You were, therefore, taught by people who did not understand the examination you were meant to take and, therefore, could not prepare you adequately for it. This resulted in your failure at the examination. It could be that the person who was sponsoring you died and there was no one to continue to bear the financial burden of your education. You were, therefore, forced to start working without attaining your academic goal. It could be that all the outward circumstances were alright and you studied hard. However, you soon found that your brain could not stand the test. You seemed to forget what you read just a few minutes afterwards. It could be that you were very brilliant, but sickness came along and you could not continue with your studies.

Whatever circumstance or event was operative, you did not attain your desired goal. As you look around, you see your classmates with the qualifications you had desired and still do. You may even see people who were not as bright as you were with the cherished diplomas. They are better qualified than you. You are disappointed with yourself. You feel frustrated. You are hurt. To make things worse, one of your "inferiors" is now your boss!

2. You did not get the job that you wanted. It could be that from childhood you very much wanted to become a medical doctor. You dreamt of the day when you would wear a spotlessly white overall, enter the theatre and carry out your first operation. You thought of the day when everyone around you would call you, "Doctor," and depend on you for their very lives. However, things did not work out that way. You failed the "A" levels. Or, you failed the entrance examination for Medical School. You then said, "I will try and become a doctor in science. In that way, I will have the coveted title, 'Doctor.'" You enrolled in the Faculty of Science and after two miserable years there, you lost your place, having failed the four major examinations in the first year . You then decided to change Faculties. You enrolled in the Faculty of Letters and even then you repeated each year, finally narrowly obtaining a degree in letters after six years in the Faculty. You are now working in an office, looking at files that do not interest you. You are disgruntled. You inwardly wish you were a doctor. Sometimes you daydream and see yourself in a white overall, attending to the sick. When you realize that you were only daydreaming you are angry with yourself.

Or, it could be that you are very well qualified for the job you desired. However, the job was given to someone who is not as qualified as you are. Or, you are due promotion. Because of corruption, you are not given the desired and well-deserved promotion. Another person is promoted and everything is done to ridicule you. Your bosses are your inferiors in every way. You feel hurt and insulted. The progress chart that you had mapped out for yourself has fallen to bits! You do not seem to see clearly any more.

3. You loved someone and wanted him to become your friend, but he chose to be the friend of another and you feel hurt. You loved someone and wanted to marry the person. At the beginning, things seemed to be going on well. Suddenly, you found that she was no longer interested. She had found someone whom she preferred. You are disappointed. You look at her new choice and, although he does not seem to be better than you, you are jealous. You say to

yourself, "I am more handsome, more educated and in every way better than he is. Why does she not prefer me?" Yes, you seem to have everything and yet you have to face the fact that, in the final analysis, your handsome looks, better education and everything else, need proving to her. You have been left aside and another person chosen.

It could be that, before you were married, your fiancé made you feel like a queen. However, after marriage, he does not care any more. No woman has drawn his attention. All you know is that you do not mean much to him any more. His career, children, car, etc, now mean more to him than you. To make things worse, when you get into his presence you seem to irritate him. He is happier alone. Before, he shared everything with you. Now, he says nothing to you. You look at yourself in the mirror. You are still beautiful. You look at your character. Much has changed for the better. You are perplexed. Before, he loved thin women. You are thin, but he says that you have become a "sack of bones." The dress he used to admire you in is now considered old-fashioned. It could be that everything you do now receives a negative comment: your capacity to handle the children, the finances of the home, the cooking, etc. You are disappointed. You feel rejected. You ask yourself, "Is this me?"

4. Another possible cause for disappointment is that the big event came but did not bring the expected glamour. You might have thought that it would be wonderful to have a degree. You worked hard for it and dreamt about it. Then the 'big' day finally came. You passed your final examination and your degree was awarded to you. However, you felt disappointed. The great feeling that you thought would come with the degree was absent. You felt empty instead. The degree did not seem to mean much to you any more. Or you thought that when you got married, you would feel on top of everything and everyone. You loved your fiancée. You laboured to win her hand and to pay all the money that was required by her parents. You arranged for a big wedding party. You bought her the most luxurious and expensive

wedding dress that you could afford. You invested much money into the feast. Then it was soon over and one week after the wedding, you felt cheated. Yes, you had her whom you loved but you did not find anything in marriage. She seemed to mean less to you after the wedding than she did before it. Many times, you have wished you were not married so that you could just be alone. It is not that your wife has failed in any way. It is just that the whole thing has turned out to be so ordinary that you wonder whether it was worth all the trouble.

A young man went out with a friend three days after he was married. The friend was asked, "Are you married?" He replied, "No." The young man who had got married three days earlier said loudly, "I wish I were you." He was disappointed.

Another young man whom I know very well said to me two weeks after his wedding, "I wish people knew that there is nothing special in marriage." Before his wedding, he could have set the whole fellowship on fire with insistence that he be allowed to be married quickly, but soon after the event he was more or less disappointed. The big event had come but failed to bring the expected glamour.

It could be that you very much wanted to preach. You prepared your sermon everyday. You were impatient with the leaders for not giving you the opportunity to preach. You waited long and, finally, the day came when you had to preach. You mounted the pulpit and began to speak. Suddenly, you found that what you were saying did not interest the audience. It did not even interest you. As you left the pulpit, you were frustrated. Many questions came into your mind: "Had you said anything reasonable? Is this all there is to preaching?" Yes, the big event had come but failed to produce the expected impact!

Maybe you thought you desperately needed a car. You would say to yourself, "When I shall buy a car, all my problems shall be solved." You planned for the car. You saved money for it and, finally, the day came when you were to have your car. Your heart was beating as you went to collect it. You brought it home, packed it outside and went to sleep. The next day you looked at it. It was there. It was yours. However, you were not too sure that it was worth all the trouble. You began to wonder whether you were not happier without it. You had gotten what you wanted, but it had failed to bring any lasting satisfaction!

It could be that you dreamt about the day you would build a house of your own. You planned well for it. You worked hard at the project, and then the house was finished. Excitedly, you went into it. There was much more room in it than in the previous house where you lived as a tenant. However, after a few days in your personal house, you found that all the excitement was gone. You also found that your deeper problems remained the same, even though you had changed houses. You feel cheated and ask, "Was there any reason for all my anxiety and all my labour?" You are disappointed!

5. Another possible cause for disappointment is in the spiritual realm. It could be that you have asked God for something over and over. You have prayed. You have petitioned. You have fasted. You have done all that you could do as an individual. Then you sought the company of another believer and together you agreed on earth concerning that thing and together asked God for it. Finally, you brought it up in the assembly and the brethren prayed and believed with you. However, the request would not be granted. You ask other things of the Lord and He gives, you. So you analyze as follows: "If God were not answering me because of some sin, why should He answer my other prayers? Why should I have peace in my relationship with Him?" You are, therefore, perplexed. You are disappointed with the promises in the Word that encourage you to ask and you will receive. It is as if heaven was sealed against you as far as that particular thing is concerned. You are disappointed with God. You ask God a question in anger, "Lord, have You ceased to be the Lord of heaven? Have You ceased to be the One who answers prayers?" You are disappointed with God. You know that He is well able to give you the

things that you have asked, but you find out that He does not seem to be doing something in that direction. You may express your disappointments in polished religious language that hides the disappointment that is deep within, but if you were true to yourself you would say, "I am disappointed with the Lord."

6. Your disappointment may come in the area of spiritual ministry. You might have invested much time, effort, prayer, etc, on some believers. You had great hopes that they would become great men of God. Then to your shock and disappointment, they turned away, one after another from following the Lord and you feel like the apostle Paul who wrote, *"Do your best to come to me soon. For Demas, in love with this present world, has deserted me and gone to Thessalonica"* (11 Timothy 4:9-10).

It could be that God gave you a vision for a ministry that would spread out to other places and bring blessings to many. You have been faithful to Him. You have worked hard at seeing the vision materialize. You have poured all of yourself into it and things have taken off the ground and you now have a clear sense of direction as to how things should proceed. You begin to visualize all the vision materialize. You are even open to further expansion, should the Lord so lead. Your co-workers are men and women of prayer and sacrifice. All seems to be going on well. Then, suddenly, the doors are shut against you. You can no longer preach the gospel publicly. You do not understand. You were working at the command of the Lord. You were working for the glory of the Lord. You examine yourself and, to the best of your knowledge, your motives for the work are pure and Christ-centred. You know that the Lord wants the gospel to reach out to many people. He is able to destroy all the barriers. You know that His Word says, *"The Lord brings the counsel of the nations to naught; he frustrates the plans of the peoples. The counsel of the Lord stands for ever, the thoughts of his heart to all generations"* (Psalm 33:10-11). However, He does nothing about the ministry, at least, not for the moment, and you feel frustrated and wonder if you have laboured in vain.

7. Another cause of disappointments is unrealistic dreams, goals or ambitions. Most people in the world fall into the following classes:

1 Those who have no goals at all.
2 Those who have vague goals.
3 Those who have clear goals that are too unambitious.
4 Those who have clear goals that are too ambitious.

Of these four classes, those who have no goals at all will not be disappointed. They set out to go nowhere. Their goal is "zero" and so they accomplish it effortlessly and have no disappointments. Those who have vague goals - goals that are not clearly thought out and written down - soon forget their momentary thoughts and do not know disappointments. Those who have unambitious goals realize these goals without much effort and, therefore, know no disappointments. Those whose goals are too ambitious often fail to realize their goals and are deeply disappointed.

PART THREE

God's answers to disappointments 1

If we want to find solutions to the problem of disappointments, we will have to find answers that God provides and put aside the answers that are offered by man. We will have to look at what God is doing, and place ourselves on His side.

GOD ALLOWS DISAPPOINTMENTS

There is no disappointment that comes to anyone who is a child of the Lord, which is not allowed or permitted by the Lord. The devil and all his agents may originate the events that lead to the disappointment, but the devil cannot touch anyone of God's children without the expressed permission of God. The devil afflicted Job. The Bible says, *"Now there was a day when his sons and daughters were eating and drinking wine in their eldest brother's house; and there came a messenger to Job, and said, 'The oxen were ploughing and the asses feeding beside them; and the Sabeans fell upon them and took them, and slew the servants with the edge of the sword; and I alone have escaped to tell you.' While he was yet speaking, there came another, and said, 'The fire of God fell from heaven and burned up the sheep and the servants, and consumed them; and I alone have escaped to tell you.' While he was yet speaking there came another, and said, 'The Chaldeans formed three companies, and made a raid upon the camels and took them, and slew the servants with the edge of the sword; and I alone have escaped to tell you.' While he was yet speaking, there came another, and said, 'Your sons and daughters were eating and drinking wine in their eldest brother's house; and behold, a great wind came across the wilderness, and struck the four corners of the house, and it fell upon the young people, and they are dead; and I alone have escaped to tell you.'*

Then Job arose, and rent his robe, and shaved his head, and fell upon the ground, and worshipped. And he said, 'Naked I came from my mother's womb, and naked shall I return; the Lord gave and the Lord has taken away; blessed be the name of the Lord.' In all this Job did not sin or charge God with wrong" (Job 1:13-22).

God permitted all this to happen to Job. The devil did it all, but he only acted because he had received permission from the Lord. The Bible says, *"Now there was a day when the sons of God came to present themselves before the Lord, and Satan also came among them. The Lord said to Satan, 'Whence have you come?' Satan answered the Lord, 'From going to and fro on the earth, and from walking up and down on it.' And the Lord said to Satan, 'Have you considered my servant Job, that there is none like him on the earth, a blameless and upright man, who fears God and turns away from evil?' Then Satan answered the Lord, 'Does Job fear God for naught? Hast thou not put a hedge about him and his house and all that he has, on every side? Thou hast blessed the work of his hands, and his possessions have increased in the land. But put forth thy hand now, and touch all that he has, and he will curse thee to thy face.' And the Lord said to Satan, 'Behold, all that he has is in your power; only upon himself do not put forth your hand.' So Satan went forth from the presence of the Lord"* (Job 1:6-12).

We see very clearly that God permitted Satan to do all that he did on Job. The Lord said to Satan, "Behold, all that he has is in your power; only upon himself do not put forth your hand." The Lord God, thus, permitted Satan to use all of his (Satan's) power against all of Job's property and children. The Lord also determined the limit within which Satan was authorized to attack. All Satan's power was allowed to go against all else that was his. Satan did that. He attacked all that Job had mercilessly and he attacked it in one day. His destruction was complete, but Job's body was not touched. In fact, regardless of how much Satan would have loved to attack Job's body, he could not. He had no permission in that direction. All his angels, demons, princes, powers and principalities with their total hatred for Job, could not touch Job at any point where the Lord gave Satan no permission. We see this illustrated further in the life of Job.

Job was steadfast after the loss of his property and children. He fell to the ground and he worshipped. He recognized that he came into the world naked and would return naked. He recognized that, although the devil was working, the devil was not final. He was not in the devil's hand. He was not controlled by the devil. He recognized the fact that the Lord permitted it. He said, "The Lord gave, and the Lord has taken away; blessed be the name of the Lord." Because he saw the hand of the Lord that permitted the devil to act, he blessed the Lord who permitted it. He did not sin or charge God with wrong.

The Bible says, *"Again there was a day when the sons of God came to present themselves before the Lord, and Satan also came among them to present himself before the Lord. And the Lord said to Satan, 'Whence have you come?' Satan answered the Lord, 'From going to and fro on the earth, and from walking up and down on it.' And the Lord said to Satan, 'Have you considered my servant Job, that there is none like him on the earth, a blameless and upright man, who fears God and turns away from evil? He will hold fast his integrity, although you moved me against him, to destroy him without cause.' Then Satan answered the Lord, 'Skin for skin! All that a man has he will give for his life. But put forth thy hand now, and touch his bone and his flesh, and he will curse thee to thy face.' And the Lord said to Satan, 'Behold, he is in your power; only spare his life.' So Satan went forth from the presence of the Lord, and afflicted Job with loathsome sores from the sole of his foot to the crown of his head. And he took a potsherd with which to scrape himself, and sat among the ashes. Then his wife said to him, 'Do you still hold fast your integrity? Curse God, and die.' But he said to her, 'You speak as one of the foolish women would speak. Shall we receive good at the hand of God, and shall we not receive evil?' In all this Job did not sin with his lips"* (Job 2:1-10).

Again, we see that Satan only acted with permission from God. We also see that he only acted within the limits that God laid down. He did not overstep those limits. He cannot overstep those limits. He is subject to God. He is not God.

TO WHOM DID GOD ALLOW DISAPPOINTMENT?

Job was not a man living actively in sin whom God used the devil to punish. On the contrary, the Bible says of him, *"And when the days of the feast had run their course, Job would send and sanctify them, and he would rise early in the morning and offer burnt offerings according to the number of them all; for Job said, 'It may be that my sons have sinned, and cursed God in their hearts.' Thus Job did continually"* (Job 1:5). The Lord Himself testified twice of Job in the following words, "There is none like him on the earth, a blameless and upright man, who fears God and turns away from evil."

Job also walked with God in the integrity of his heart. He spoke out of a clear conscience before the Lord and said, *"I have made a covenant with my eyes; how then could I look upon a virgin? What would be my portion from God above, and my heritage from the Almighty on high?"* (Job 31:1-2). He further said, *"If my heart has been enticed to a woman, and I have lain in wait at my neighbour's door; then let my wife grind for another, and let others bow down upon her"* (Job 31:9-10). Job was pure in all aspects of the sexual life. Again he said, *"If I have walked with falsehood, and my foot has hastened to deceit; (Let me be weighed in a just balance, and let God know my integrity!) if my step has turned aside from the way, and my heart has gone after my eyes, and if any spot has cleaved to my hands; then let me sow, and another eat; and let what grows for me be rooted out"* (Job 31:5-8). Job was without falsehood and without greed. He also was just with his servants (Job 31:13). He gave to the poor (Job 31:16-23). He was without the love of money (Job 31:24-25). He loved his enemies (Job 31:29-32). He exposed his sin and had been delivered from the opinion of men (Job 31:33-35). Job was really an upright man. Yet he is the one whom God allowed Satan to inflict. Why was that so?

GOD'S USE OF DISAPPOINTMENT

The Lord had said of Job before his troubles began, " .... that there is none like him on earth, a blameless and upright man, who fears God and turns away from evil." This was very recommendable. Job had made much progress in holiness. He was submissive to the will of God, but he was not completely perfect. He had not reached the highest standard of maturity. He knew God, but his knowledge of God had not yet reached the ultimate point. He said after his suffering, *"I had heard of thee by the hearing of the ear, but now my eye sees thee; therefore I despise myself, and repent in dust and ashes"* (Job 42:5-6). Through suffering he passed from the state of "hearing" of God to that of "seeing" God. He passed from the man who spoke freely about his righteousness in all domains of life to one who despised himself, repented and was humble.

The disappointment of Job, which was the work of Satan in the permissive will of God, became God's appointment with Job to bring him to spiritual maturity. He became a man who did not accept the sovereign will of God by resignation, but one who accepted it joyfully, even after suffering, saying, *"I know that thou canst do all things, and that no purpose of thine can be thwarted"* (Job 42:2). God had purposed to bring Job to perfection. He had found in him a willing man who did not cling to what he had. In that union of a righteous man, who was not yet perfect, and a perfect God, the Lord used the instruments of suffering, affliction, etc, to produce a man after His own heart in every way.

Man's disappointments are God's appointments. The one who sees this divine truth will welcome every disappointment with joy, for it is God's appointment. The Bible says, "We know that in everything God works for good with those who love him, who are called according to his purpose" (Romans 8:28). Do you see what the word of God is saying? Do you see what God is saying? That His disappointments are for your good - if you love Him and are called according to His purpose. This being true, there is only one thing that a believer needs to do. He needs to ensure that he loves the Lord and is called according to God's purpose. When he is sure of that, he can be perfectly at rest; for all that comes to him will be used by God for his good. Disappointments may come, failures may come, enemies may come, doors may be closed, promotions may be hindered, rejections may come, difficulties may come, betrayals may come, persecutions may come, all kinds of situations may come. However, in each one of them and for all of them together, God will work for the good of that believer who loves Him and is called according to His purpose. The believer who loves the Lord and is called according to God's purpose does not worry about who is planning what against him. He knows that nothing will happen to him that his loving heavenly Father has not permitted. He also knows that in all that the Lord will permit, He will also work for his good.

There is no possibility that Satan can bypass the Lord and get at the believer who loves the Lord and is called according to His purpose. There is no possibility that Satan can prevent the Lord from working in everything and in every situation for the good of the believer who loves the Lord and is called according to His purpose. The Bible says,

"The Lord brings the counsel of the nations to nought; he frustrates the plans of the peoples.
The counsel of the Lord stands for ever, the thoughts of his heart to all generations" (Psalm 33:10-11).

The Lord will bring all the counsel of the nations to nought. He will frustrate all the plans of the devil and the plans of man which He cannot use to bless those who love Him and are called according to His purpose. His counsel, which includes the fact that He will work in all things for good for those who love Him and are called according to His purpose, stands for evermore. His thoughts, which include that of working in everything for the good of those who love Him and are called according to His purpose, stand for ever.

Alec Brooks* put it this way, "God does not cause everything to happen, but He rules over everything. His sovereignty is such that He is able to use whatever occurs. He weaves each event into His great purpose for us, no matter what anyone else may intend. When our trust is in God, everything is filtered through His love, and if we will trust Him, it will produce good. Satan is frustrated by the lives of those who trust God. Not only is he unable to harm them, but everything negative he does toward them becomes positive in their lives."

Joseph was sold by his brothers. He suffered imprisonment in Egypt. He later on became the governor of Egypt under Pharaoh. He told his brethren who had maltreated him, *"As for you, you meant evil against me; but God meant it for good, to bring it about that many people should be kept alive, as they are today"* (Genesis 50:20). His brothers meant him evil, but God meant good for him through this act of evil by his brothers. In the end we see, not the evil intentions of his brothers prevailing, but the good that God intended. Yes, "The counsel of the Lord stands for ever, the thoughts of his heart to all generations." The Lord of hosts has sworn, *"As I have planned, so shall it be, and as I have purposed, so shall it stand"* (Isaiah 14:24).

So God will use your disappointment, regardless of what it is, for your good, provided you love Him and are called according to His purpose. Your disappointments are His appointments.

If you do not love Him and are not called according to His purpose, He wants to use your disappointments to bring you to love Him and be called according to His purpose. Could anything be better for you?

PART FOUR

God's answers to disappointments 2

We have seen that God will work in everything for the good of those who love Him and are called according to His purpose. We believe that it is necessary to state clearly the purpose that God has in mind, so that there may be no misunderstanding.

Many think that God's purpose is that things should move smoothly and painlessly and that they should have the maximum enjoyment at no cost to themselves. Some believers think that it is God's will that the believer should be rich, have plenty of things, live in undisturbed luxury, be loved and respected by everyone. God can bring these things to the believer, and He sometimes does. However, God will not work in everything for the good of the believer so that he should live at ease,

gaiety,
acceptance,
etc.

God will not work in everything for the good of the believer so that he is first in his class,

never fails an examination,
is promoted to the top of his career,
has all his wants supplied, has perfect harmony at his job site,
home, etc.

God will work in everything for good for the one who loves Him and is called according to His purpose, so that that one may be *"CONFORMED TO THE IMAGE OF HIS SON, IN ORDER THAT HE MIGHT BE THE FIRST-BORN AMONG MANY BRETHREN"* (Romans 8:29). The purpose of God is that His adopted sons should conform to the image of His only begotten Son in everything. God will work in all things to ensure that His adopted sons conform to His only begotten Son.

If that is God's goal, then those who are going to conform to the

Lord Jesus will know very many disappointments. Why is this so? It has to be so because many people do not know what it means to come to the Lord Jesus, or they are mistaken about what coming to Jesus means. Jesus said, *"If any man would come after me, let him deny himself and take up his cross daily and follow me"* (Luke 9:23). This is the first lesson in the christian life. The Bible again says, *"Do not love the world or the things in the world. If anyone loves the world, love for the Father is not in him. For all that is in the world, the lust of the flesh and the lust of the eyes and the pride of life, is not of the Father but is of the world. And the world passes away, and the lust of it; but he who does the will of God abides for ever"* (1 John 2:15-17).

If God's will is that all His should deny themselves, take up their crosses daily and follow Him to that place where the self-life is crucified, to that place where the desire to be loved, appreciated and honoured is put to death, to that place where the love of the world and the love of the things of the world is crucified, then He will of necessity disappoint very many in their natural desires, and these disappointments will be His appointments.

Let us look at the disappointments that we listed out in chapter one and see if the initial desires were for the glory of God or for the glory of self. If a person did not get the education he would have loved to have for himself and is disappointed, we may ask why he wanted that education. Was it not so that his self-importance might be enhanced? Was it solely for God's glory with nothing of "self" in it? Was it God's will for him? Was that education absolutely necessary to make him conform to the Lord Jesus in all things? Was it not good that God should allow him to be disappointed in his selfish desires so that that God might re-appoint him along His one purpose for him, which is, conformity to the Lord Jesus in all things? Ought he not have said, "Lord, thank You for allowing me to be disappointed on the road of self-seeking and for appointing me on the way of being like Christ"?

When a person does not get the job he wanted but is given another job by the Lord and he is disappointed because he did not get the job of his first choice, is it not obvious that he wanted that job for self-glory and not for God's glory? Out of love for him, should the Lord not allow him to be disappointed along his path of self-seeking, so that He may re-appoint him on God's chosen path for him, which is, seeking to be like the Lord Jesus? Was Jesus not the King of heaven? Did He not spend most of His earthly life as a carpenter? Did He despise that job or did He do it faithfully?

When someone's love is not reciprocated and he feels disappointed and hurt, the question can be asked whether it was love at all or whether it was a selfish desire to have the other person related to him. True love seeks to give and give and give. It does not seek to receive. It does not seek response; for that is self. The one who truly loves, gives and gives and finds perfect satisfaction in giving. If the person who is loved responds, he continues to give. If he does not respond, he continues to give. Because he loves (and no one can love until he is delivered from self), he thinks of the welfare of the loved one and rejoices with the loved one, even if the loved one finds fulfilment, not in loving him, but in loving another. The truth is that what most people call love is self-love. It dies when it is not responded to. It seeks the attention of another and wants to receive. When nothing or too little is given in return, it is hurt and dies.

Since the purpose of God is to deliver us from self and especially from self-love, will it not be a wonderful thing when God works out so that our self-love, which we thought was love for someone, is hurt, when, through that process, we are delivered from self-love and can begin to love the person in truth, regardless of the response we receive?

When the big event comes but does not bring the expected glamour, does that not show that joy and happiness are being sought or expected from that which is ephemeral? The Bible says that the world passes away and the lust thereof. When God allows such a disappointment, ought the believer not to thank Him for taking the shadow on which he was concentrating so that he might concentrate on the Lord Jesus, who is the real substance? Why should degrees, marriages and preaching be made the goals of life? Are these not the goals of worldly men? Is it not an act of love when God uses disappointments to open our eyes? Have your eyes been opened since you were disappointed? Have you repented or have you made another shadow your goal to replace the one that disappointed you?

When your disappointment comes in the realm of spiritual ministry, do you not see that it is possibly God's way to prune you who are already bearing fruit, so that you may bear more fruit? The Lord Jesus said, *"I am the true vine, and my father is the vinedresser. Every branch of mine that bears no fruit, he takes away, and every branch that does bear fruit he prunes, that it may bear more fruit"* (John 15:1-2). If the disappointment came because you were mistaken about God's will, ought you not to thank the Lord for loving you so much that He has not allowed you to labour in vain? For, does He not say that every plant which His heavenly Father has not planted will be uprooted? Was it not good that it should be stopped now, rather than that you should invest many years in it, only to find, in the end, that it was all wood, hay and stubble? Is it not a blessing that you should at least use the rest of your time seeking God's will and doing it, so that there will be something to your credit on that Day? Ought you not to thank God for the disappointment and receive it with joy? God always accomplishes His purpose. If He allows something to be stopped now, does that not say that He wants something else for now? Why should anyone want anything, however glorious it may appear, that God does not want? Is that not utter rebellion to want that which God does not want?

When a person sets goals that are unrealistic, is it not obvious that these goals originated in "self" and not in the Lord? Does it not mean that he did not wait on God enough in order to receive God's goals and to work at them? When God allows a man's selfish goals to crumble, is it not a sign of love? Should the person not then praise and thank the Lord and move in the direction of seeking God's will and doing it?

God wants His adopted sons to conform to the only begotten Son in all things. He will use disappointments and all else that are necessary to accomplish that goal. Those who love Him more will be closer to Him. They will also receive more discipline from Him, because He will correct them to a greater extent than He will do with those who love Him only a little.

Each disappointment tells us there is a flaw which He wants to take away. The apostle Paul knew much of it. He said, *"And to keep me from being too elated by the abundance of revelations, a thorn was given me in the flesh, a messenger of Satan, to harass me, to keep me from being too elated. Three times I besought the Lord about this, that it should leave me; but he said to me, 'My grace is sufficient for you, for my power is made perfect in weakness.' I will all the more gladly boast of my weaknesses, that the power of Christ may rest upon me. For the sake of Christ, then, I am content with weaknesses, insults, hardships, persecutions, and calamities; for when I am weak, then I am strong"* (2 Corinthians 12:7-10).

Are you prepared to be content with weaknesses, hardships,
persecutions,
calamities,
insults, etc.,

so that when you are weak you may be made strong in the Lord? Are you prepared to have all your natural strength and ability brought to nought, so that you may receive the supernatural strength and ability of Christ?

To have weaknesses, that is, the inability to do anything on your own (and in your own strength), having to depend on the Lord for everything, is true spirituality. It is true contentment. It is the way of faith. It is the life that pleases God. It is the way of death to self. It is the way of life in Christ. It is the way of inner healing. It is the way of inner health. It is the way for those who want only one thing -

total conformity to the Lord Jesus in everything. Such people are winners. They are the healed, the healthy!

God has an eternal view of things. When He works in the believer, it is not for temporary good, but for eternal good. Some things may appear very bad on the temporary scale of time, but when viewed from eternity they are excellent. The Bible says, *"For the moment all discipline seems painful rather than pleasant; later it yields the peaceful fruit of righteousness to those who have been trained by it"* (Hebrews 12:11). The apostle Paul said, *"For this slight momentary affliction is preparing for us an eternal weight of glory beyond all comparison, because we look not to the things that are seen but to the things that are unseen; for the things that are seen are transient, but the things that are unseen are eternal"* (2 Corinthians 4:17-18).

Those who ask in each situation what the eternal consequences of each action are, will be delivered from fretting over temporary consequences, and enter into the rest of the God who sees all things from an eternal perspective and is not preoccupied with the passing.

From the eternal perspective, suffering, persecution, poverty, self-denial, etc, take on a new importance, because they become instruments in God's hands for building the quality of character that will fit those who are to reign with the Lord in His kingdom. Those who see things from God's eternal perspective enter into rest now!

PART FIVE

Guilt and inner healing

A girl was born in a christian family. Early in life she gave her life to the Lord Jesus. Her parents walked with God and the moral standards of the home were high. She was taught clearly that sexual immorality was not only the sexual act but, as the Lord Jesus put it, *"Everyone who looks at a woman lustfully has already committed adultery with her in his heart"* (Matthew 5:28). She was, therefore, brought up to know that premarital kissing,

petting,
caressing,
etc,

was sinful before the Lord. They constituted fornication in the heart. At the age of eighteen she got engaged. She was still a virgin and had never indulged in any kissing, petting, caressing or reading of immoral books. During the period of their engagement, which lasted two years, her fiancé, whose spiritual commitment and standard of holiness were lower, insisted on kissing and petting, which became increasingly intense. Although she gave in to it reluctantly at first, she later on took the initiative to encourage him. She calmed her conscience that was accusing her and thought it was alright. She would sometimes tell herself that her thoughts had remained pure even when the caressing was going on. Occasionally, she asked God to forgive her and promised never to allow it to happen again, but the next time when they met, it would still happen. On the night of their wedding, she was most unresponsive. The marriage was not consummated until the third day, when the man literally "raped" her. Throughout the marriage, she hardly found any fulfilment in the marital relationship. She hated herself and she hated her husband. Each time the husband came in from work, the thought immediately came up to her. "This is the man who caused you to commit the sin of fornication, even though you were physically a virgin." Another thought would come up to her, "You are a cheap and useless woman. You allowed your body to be touched all over before marriage." As these thoughts came up, she would close herself up and hate him and herself. This meant that all areas of their marriage life were affected, not just the sexual. She was suffering from guilt. She was sick of guilt.

There are many people whose problem of inner healing is associated with guilt. It does not matter what the sin committed may be. Sin is the breaking of God's law, and God's law has the force of a physical law and more. No one can commit sin and just continue living normally. All sin that is committed destroys the personality of the one who commits it to a varying extent, depending upon the light that has been received, unless the sin is well- handled. It is not a matter of saying that a sin is big or small. All sin is sin. I suffered under the weight of a "small" lie that I had told my mother at the age of twenty-nine until I was completely healed.

The problems of many people have their roots in guilt. They might have committed some sin and, as their conscience accused them, they did everything to calm their conscience and hide the sin. Or they might have carried out a false confession which still left the guilt buried deep down into their inner being, like a small cancerous cell, to multiply and cause damage in many areas of the person's life. We know that there are some venereal diseases which are manifested by an initial symptom. If the disease is not treated at that stage, the symptom disappears and everything seems fine. Later on, there are secondary symptoms which may also disappear until many years afterwards, when the tertiary symptoms like blindness, etc, show up. The person may not relate his blindness to the immoral sexual relationship that he practised years before, but that is it. He may not even know that venereal disease could result in blindness, but that will not prevent him from being blind.

Sin does not only ruin a person's relationship with God. It ruins the person. It ruins his character and it ruins his personality. Some guilt is immediately discernable. Some is very "quiet" and some may be buried so deep that it may seem not to exist. Nevertheless, it is there and its devastating work continues until it is dealt with.

HOW TO HANDLE GUILT

The matter of handling guilt is indeed the matter of handling sin. Our first recommendation is that you should not commit sin. It is easier to keep away from sin than to handle the consequences of sin. Many of the consequences of sin cannot be brought under control by man, once the deed has been done. Two sisters committed the tragic sin of gossipping about another sister. One of the two told what the other had said to a brother, who told the story to another sister in a different town. This sister in her own turn told the story to another brother who lived in another town. As each person told the story, he or she added what he thought would make it more reasonable and more convincing, and the final story that got to me was scandalous. There is nothing that the initial gossips can ever do to undo the harm that they did to the character of the sister about whom they gossipped. A bomb was let loose that continued to devastate. So, we insist that the best way to handle guilt is never to allow it the opportunity to ever occur. The Bible says, *"Submit yourself therefore to God. Resist the devil and he will flee from you"* (James 4:7). *"Walk by the Spirit, and do not gratify the desires of the flesh"* (Galatians 5:16).

The Lord Jesus took us with Himself to the cross. Our old man was crucified with Him once and for all, so that we may not be slaves to sin but slaves to righteousness. Each believer can live without committing sin. Each believer should live without committing sin.

However, believers do commit sin and are guilty. In addition to this, there are sins that were committed before the person became a child of God. These sins also have their effect on the person. In order to handle the matter simply, we are going to handle all guilt together, regardless of whether it is for sin committed before or after the person had believed.

1. ACKNOWLEDGE THAT SIN IS SIN

There will never be true healing until the person involved acknowledges sin as sin. If he calls it a mistake, a fault, an error, etc, he is not yet prepared for healing. Acknowledging sin as sin includes calling sin by its name. The person who says, "I am not holy," instead of saying, "I committed fornication in my thoughts," is not yet ready for healing. The one who says, "I took some money away," instead of saying, "I stole some money," is not ready for healing. The person who says, "I told just part of the story," instead of saying, "I lied to him," is not yet ready for healing, etc. We insist that sin must be called by its name and things must be put clearly. The one who has committed adultery or fornication should write out how many times it has occurred and with whom. Attempts to be vague or to hide some of the sin are determined efforts to block healing, and God will not heal anyone who does not want to be healed.

At some point, it is important for the person who wants to be healed from guilt to go to a quiet place and ask God to show him all the sins he has committed but which were never really dealt with the way the Bible wants sin to be dealt with. He should carry a notebook and a pen with him. If he is honest, God will begin to show him the hidden sins of his life. I once did this and so I know it from personal experience. It was as if the film of my life was suddenly put before me. I began to see everything I had done and never truly repented of. It went on and on, year after year, event after event and I wrote the things down as I saw them. I recognized everything I saw. I was fully aware that everything I saw was known by me to be wrong when I did it or said it or refused to say it or do it. So I wrote the things down. At each step, I asked the Lord to forgive me. Even though I was seeing my unconfessed sin, the Lord made it in such a way that it was not painful, so that I was not broken when it was all over.

I am fully persuaded that the Lord will enable the sins that anyone committed but did not repent of and forsake, to be shown to him so that he may deal with them accordingly. However, the person must ask the Lord and he must ask with insistence. He must wait before the Lord so that things can be shown to him. After all, nothing is hidden from the Lord! The person should also ask with the full determination that he will deal radically with anything that the Lord shows him. Without this willingness (and the Lord knows our heart and does not just listen to our words), the Lord will show us nothing; for He does not play games.

When all the sin that the Lord wants to show us at that moment has been revealed to us and we have taken note of all, then follows the second step.

2. CONFESS ALL SIN

In the confession of sin, a person acknowledges his sin to the Lord. He has been helped by the Lord to see things as they are. He must now own up to God that the sin is his. He must not say, "We have sinned." He must say, "I have sinned." Then he must now name each sin to God, not seeking to justify any. The Bible says, *"He who conceals his transgressions will not prosper, but he who confesses and forsakes them will obtain mercy"* (Proverbs 28:13). *"When I declared not my sin, my body wasted away through my groaning all day long. For day and night thy hand was heavy upon me; my strength was dried up as by the heat of summer. I acknowledged my sin to thee, and I did not hide my iniquity; I said, 'I will confess my transgression to the Lord,' then thou didst forgive the guilt of my sin"* (Psalm 32:3-5).

It is useless to confess sin in part. It will result in no forgiveness. It is also useless to confess sin and not terminate with it radically and once and for all. God is not mocked. He cannot be deceived. He deals with the hearts of men and not just with the confessions of their lips. If anyone says to Him, "Lord, I confess this sin and that sin to you," He will not just listen to the words. He will look at the heart to see if there is hatred of that sin and of all other sins. He will look to see if there are other sins in the person's life that are known to the person but which the person has not confessed. Then He will see if the person has said a final 'good bye' to these sins in his heart. If the Lord does not see this, He will close His ears to the person's confession; for it is not confession but deceit, and God will not be deceived.

However, if He sees a departure from all sin in the heart of the person, He will receive the confession and forgive the person. The Bible says, *"If we confess our sins, he is faithful and just, and will forgive our sins and cleanse us from all unrighteousness"* (1 John 1:9). When the Lord forgives, He forgives. He does not forgive in part. His forgiveness is full and it is thorough. The Bible says, *"As far as the east is from the west, so far does he remove our transgressions from us"* (Psalm 103:12)

3. ACCEPT GOD'S FORGIVENESS

I have met people who have carried a sense of guilt for years. They have all said to me, "I know God has forgiven me but I cannot forgive myself." Many of such people are truly restless. For many of them, I found they had not truly repented and, therefore, they could not enjoy the peace of God, which comes with true repentance and forgiveness. They were only sorry about their sin. They may weep each time they think of their sin, but they have never genuinely repented. True repentance involves a change of mind, a change of heart and a change of course. Those who go back to their sin never had a change of heart and a change of course. Someone may wonder how a person can weep and be miserable for days without having repented. I have seen many weep and weep and continue as before. At one evangelistic meeting, we preached on the Samaritan woman. In the audience was a woman who had had five children with five different men, none of whom was her husband. She saw herself in the story and felt sorry for herself. She saw the problems she was having and wept. She wished things were better. She refused to repent, forsake immoral living and give her heart to the Lord. She continued to weep when she was being counselled, but they were tears of self-pity and not tears of repentance. Her eyes were blinded to the Lord whose law she had broken. She was pre-occupied with herself.

Genuine repentance implies that a person has seen his sin as committed against God. He is not, first of all, pre-occupied with the consequences of his sin on himself either in time or in eternity. He is pre-occupied with what his sin has done to the glory, honour and holiness of God. He repents for bringing such dishonour to God. He receives forgiveness from God for the evil he did to His (God's) name. With that settled, the person can then look at the secondary consequences of his sin, which include:

1. His present life.
2. His relationship with others.
3. His future after death.

If a person has truly repented towards God, he will gladly accept God's forgiveness. The barrier that stood between him and God is removed. The person will know in his heart that the Lord has forgiven him. The Holy Spirit always brings that witness to the human spirit when there is genuine repentance. This inner witness is different from the theoretical knowledge of the facts that those whose confession is spurious have. Their spurious repentance will lead to a spurious assurance of forgiveness, and the proof of the falsehood of it is that they will go back to committing the same sin. Those who genuinely repent hardly ever fall into the same sin again.

Because God has accepted the person and forgiven him, He has also taken away the eternal consequences of his sin. He will never be called to answer for it. He will never be excluded from heaven because of it. The Holy Spirit also bears witness to the spirit of the one who has genuinely repented about this. So, the person accepts himself by the witness of the Holy Spirit to his spirit and the testimony of the word of God as having eternal life.

Many people will find that they still carry guilt for sin, even after genuine repentance and true restoration by the Lord. Why is this so? It is so because the consequences of sin in time must be dealt with.

4. ACCEPT GOD'S FORGIVENESS

People who have genuinely repented and received the forgiveness of God may find that they still carry a sense of guilt. This is not because of their Godward relationship, but because of their manward relationship. Because the manward affects the Godward, the person may lack boldness before God.

To avoid this kind of situation, a person should carry out restitution. He has put things right with God. He should put things right with man. When Zacchaeus encountered the Lord Jesus, he said, *"Behold, Lord, the half of my goods I give to the poor; and if I have defrauded anyone of anything, I restore it fourfold"* (Luke 19:8). He was acting on an Old Testament precept that said, *"If anyone sins and commits a breach of faith against the Lord by deceiving his neighbour in a matter of deposit or security, or through robbery, or if he has oppressed his neighbour or has found what was lost and lied about it, swearing falsely - in any of all the things which men do and sin therein, when one has sinned and become guilty, he shall restore what he took by robbery, or what he got by oppression, or the deposit which was committed to him, or the lost thing which he found, or anything about which he has sworn falsely; he shall restore it in full, and shall add a fifth to it, and give it to him to whom it belongs, on the day of his guilt offering. And he shall bring to the priest his guilt offering to the Lord, a ram without blemish out of the flock, valued by you at the price for a guilt offering; and the priest shall make atonement for him before the Lord, and he shall be forgiven for any of the things which one may do and thereby become guilty"* (Leviticus 6:2-7).

"For every breach of trust, whether it is for ox, for ass, for sheep, for clothing, or for any kind of lost thing, of which one says, 'This is it,' the case of both parties shall come before God; he whom God shall condemn shall pay double to his neighbour" (Exodus 22:9). *"If a man steals an ox or a sheep, and kills it or sells it, he shall pay five oxen for an ox, and four sheep*

for a sheep. He shall make restitution; if he has nothing, then he shall be sold for his theft. If the stolen beast is found alive in his possession, whether it is an ox or an ass or a sheep, he shall pay double" (Exodus 22:1-4).

Restitution has to be deep and thorough. Lies have to be confessed, false words, attitudes, relationships, etc, have to be confessed to man after they have been confessed to God. Misplaced affections and ambitions have to be confessed and put right. Jealousies, rivalries, etc, have to be confessed and forsaken. Stolen goods of all kinds have to be confessed and restitution carried out. False confessions of love, friendship, loyalty, etc.... have to be confessed to the parties that were deceived. Gossips have to be confessed to the parties concerned. The confessions will need to be deep and thorough and forgiveness pleaded for from the party that was wounded and from whom forgiveness is sought. In asking for forgiveness, a person should not just be seeking to ease his conscience. He should labour to heal the wounds that were caused by his sin or sins. So, it is not just a matter of asking for forgiveness. It includes a labour to impart healing where hurt was caused. So, the one asking for forgiveness has to plead for it. He will have to pray that God should touch the one he hurt and grant him the grace to forgive him. He will, therefore, pray before going to confess whatever has to be confessed and, afterwards, he has to pray that the Lord should heal the wounds that he caused. The purpose will be to bring the person who was deceived or defrauded to a position that is as much as possible what it would have been had he not been wronged. For example, the father of an illegitimate child will carry out restitution by caring for the mother of the child materially and in all ways in all purity until she no longer needs him. He will also take care of the illegitimate child for as long as the child will need him. A person who gossipped and caused the character of another to be assassinated will be prepared to go to as many people as the story has gone and put things right. The same thing applies to a person who lied. He must be prepared to go as far as the lie has spread and put things right. He may have to write a circular letter or publish something in a paper owning up to his guilt and clearing the guiltless.

Restitution is not something that can be forced on anyone by another or by a religious system. The Holy Spirit and the Word convict people and tell them what they should do. I suggest that each believer should take time before the Lord and ask him, "Where do I need to carry out restitution?" The Lord will speak to him and show him what he must do and how he must do it. In the past, we discussed restitution with people who came for counselling and suggested to them what they should do. I feel most reluctant to carry out that type of counselling now. I prefer to let a person deal directly with the Lord who lives in him, listen to Him, hear Him, obey Him and face the consequences with Him or disobey Him and face the consequences before Him. There are deep issues involved in restitution that only the Holy Spirit can sort out with the person concerned. We can trust Him to deal with the honest heart accordingly. We can also trust Him to know to what extent to strive with those who do not want to carry out the restitution that He is demanding.

When restitution is not carried out as the Holy Spirit demands, the person may go on as if he were normal. It may be that he does not carry a feeling of guilt, but his Christian walk and his character will be affected in one way or another. He may have constant problems in one area of his life without knowing that the root cause stems from the restitution he refused to carry out.

Because all areas of a person's character and personality are related and, because problems in one area may cause manifestations in another, anyone who wants total inner healing and the fullness of Christ must ensure that he obeys the Holy Spirit promptly in all the things that He has shown and is showing him. He must constantly ask him, "Lord, am I hiding sin anywhere in my life? If so, show me." He must plead with the Lord to show him if there is anything wrong. If anything is shown to him, he must deal with it thoroughly, regardless of what it will cost him.

There will be areas of restitution that the Lord will not show the believer at the beginning of his Christian walk, but which He will show him later on when he has made some progress and is able to handle things better. This means that even though a person faced his sin and carried out very thorough restitution at the beginning of his Christian walk or later on, he should not consider that he has settled the matter of restitution once and for all. He can only say that to the present moment he has obeyed the Lord (that is if he has indeed obeyed the Lord) to the extent to which the Lord has shown him things. He should continue to seek more light from the Lord, and if other things are shown to him for which restitution should be carried out, he should confess them and carry out restitution and, in this way, remain in the current of the Holy Spirit, in physical health and inner health.

Amen.

PART SIX

The sins of parents and inner healing

Read the following; "Max Jules, the atheist, lived a godless life. He married an ungodly girl. From that union the following were produced:

310 paupers,
150 criminals,
7 murderers,
100 drunkards,

More than half of the women were prostitutes. His 540 known descendants cost the United States government 1,250,000 dollars."

Jonathan Edward (a leading revivalist) lived at the same time with atheist Max Jules. He married a godly girl. An investigation was made of his 1,394 known descendants:-

13 became college presidents,
66 became college professors (University teachers).
3 became United States Senators,
30 became judges,
100 became lawyers,
60 became medical doctors,
75 became army and navy officers,
100 became preachers and missionaries,
60 became authors of prominence,
1 became a Vice-President of the United States of America,
80 became public officers in other capacities,
295 became University graduates among whom were state governors, United States Representatives to foreign countries, etc.

None of his descendants cost the United States government a cent." (Quoted from the book, "Meat for Men" by L. Ravenhill).

People suffer from the consequences of their sin. They also suffer for the sins of their parents, grandparents and great grandparents. The Lord said, *"I the Lord your God am a jealous God, visiting the iniquity of the fathers upon the children to the third and the fourth generation of those who hate me, but showing steadfast love to thousands of those who love me and keep my commandments"* (Exodus 20:5-6). *"The Lord, the Lord, a God merciful and gracious, slow to anger, and abounding in steadfast love and faithfulness, keeping steadfast love for thousands, forgiving iniquity and transgression and sin, but who will by no means clear the guilty, visiting the iniquity of the fathers upon the children and the children's children, to the third and the fourth generation"* (Exodus 34:6-7).

It is immediately obvious that the sins of our parents, grandparents and great grandparents have an effect on us. In a way that I cannot explain, children tend to do many negative things that their parents or grandparents did, even though they did not live with these people to be able to copy from them. There are characteristics that are transmitted from parents to children in a way that modern genetics does not explain. For example, it has been observed that selfishness, immorality, dishonesty, etc, can be traced in a family up to the fourth generation and beyond. We know that there are entire tribes that are bound by the love of money or by an unforgiving spirit, yet these traits are not easily learnt or transmitted by any genetic process that we know of today. The only explanation that makes sense to me is that God has continued to keep His word and to visit the sins of the parents on the children, grandchildren and great grandchildren.

If that is so, then people are suffering from the consequences of sins that they sort of "inherited". The strange behaviour of some people may be the result of the judgment of God on them because of the sins of their ancestors. What should be done about it? It will be best to answer this question by looking at how the men of the Bible handled the matter.

A) NEHEMIAH

He prayed : *"O Lord God of heaven, the great and terrible God who keeps covenant and steadfast love with those who love Him and keep his commandments; let thy ear be attentive, and thy eyes open, to hear the prayer of thy servant which I now pray before thee day and night for the people of Israel thy servants, confessing the sins of the people of Israel, which we have sinned against thee. Yea, I and my father's house have sinned. We have acted very corruptly against thee, and have not kept the commandment, the statutes, and the ordinances which thou didst command thy servant Moses"* (Nehemiah 1:5-7).

B) DANIEL

He prayed, *"O Lord, the great and terrible God, who keepest covenant and steadfast love with those who love him and keep his commandments, we have sinned and done wrong and acted wickedly and rebelled, turning aside from thy commandments and ordinances; we have not listened to thy servants the prophets, who spoke in thy name to our kings, our princes, and our fathers, and to all the people of the land .... "* (Daniel 9:4-14).

We see that these men of God took upon themselves the sins of their people and made them their own. They identified fully with the sins of their people, even though they themselves did not commit those sins. They owned them before God as theirs and pleaded with the Lord for mercy. They confessed their personal sins thoroughly and they confessed the sins of their people as thoroughly as they could.

God heard them and forgave them and their people and showed them mercy. The sins of our ancestors can be handled similarly. It does not matter whether or not they are dead. It only matters that they sinned and that the consequences of their sins and sin are upon us. This confession of sin will not get them to heaven. It is for our benefit, since we are the ones suffering from the consequences of what they did. In order to receive inner healing from problems caused by ancestry, we suggest the following procedure:

1 You should ensure that you have dealt with your personal sin and carried out restitution as thoroughly as was shown in the preceding chapter. Unless this has been done as honestly as possible, it will be useless to try and take upon yourself the sins of your ancestors. How will you honestly confess their sins when you are dishonest about your own sins?

2 You should repent of any attitude of hate or resentment for any of your ancestors that you may be harbouring. You may be an illegitimate child and feel bitter and resentful of your promiscuous mother whose sin caused you to be born under unusual circumstances, or you may be bitter and resentful of your father for making your mother pregnant and refusing to marry her. Yours could be an ancestry of drunkards, thieves, lazy people, spend thrifts, etc, and you might have been bitter against them for years. You should repent of your sin of resentment and bitterness against them for a number of reasons:

- First of all, if you continue to be bitter and resentful, you will be the one to suffer, and not they, for your resentment. Why bring that suffering on yourself?
- You will pass their sin on to your children, unless you repent and forsake it.
- You will be blocked in your communion with God because of the bitterness and resentment.
- You will soon begin to suffer physically because of your sin of bitterness and resentment.
-Etc.

3 You must accept on you all the sins of your father and mother, your grandparents and your great grandparents on your father's and mother's sides. This must not be done in a superficial way; for no superficial thing has a place in the purpose of God. You should write out all the sins of your parents that you can remember. You should find out any sins of your grandparents that you know and write them out. When you have made a list

that is as exhaustive as possible, seek a quiet place and be alone with God.

While before the Lord, take all the sins of your ancestors upon yourself. Say to the Lord, "These sins are mine; for I was in the loins of my ancestors when they committed them. I do not justify them or myself for any of the sins they committed. I make no attempt to palliate their evil doings. I acknowledge that the sins here listed are only a small portion of the total. You know them all, Lord, forgive these. Lord, forgive all the other ones. I hand over to you each one of them and all of them together and plead, Lord, that you should take all of them away because they were taken by the Lord Jesus with Him to His victorious death. Do it now, Lord. Amen".

4 You should release all those who are alive and who are suffering because God has visited these sins upon them. It is better to call people by name. Ask the Holy Spirit to show you anyone who is held captive because of the sins of the ancestors. He will show you. He will even show you what part of the person's personality is held in bondage. As He shows you the people and the areas in which they are held captive, unbind them in the name of the Lord. Say, "In the name of the Lord Jesus, I release .... from the bondage to... that was caused by the sins of his ancestors. I break the power of this bondage and set him free once and for all. In the name of Jesus, I bring to an end, once and for all, all tendencies to have this evil perpetrated in the future. Amen." Having ministered to each one in this way, you should now minister to yourself. You may know some abnormalities in your character or personality that you cannot explain. There may be things in your own behaviour which are totally out of tune with the rest of your person and conduct. These may be due to the sins of your ancestors being visited upon you. Confess all such sins. Lift up to the Lord each abnormal attitude and ask the Lord to take it away. Lay all those abnormalities on the Lord and refuse to take them upon your-

self any more. Believe that the Lord has dealt away with them. Ask the Lord to take away any consequences of these upon any of your relatives or children, and stand on victory ground for yourself and for them all. The Lord is faithful. He will act accordingly. Glory be unto Him!

There is one more area which we want to deal with before we move away from this chapter. It has to do with national or tribal tendencies. We know that there are some negative characteristics that are generally associated with some nations, races or tribes. For example, some groups of people tend to be generally:

ruthless, or

unforgiving, or
lazy, or
purposeless, or
quick-tempered, or
greedy, or
vain, or
stingy, or
gluttonous, or
given to wine, or
given to pleasure, or
given to immorality, or
aggressive,
etc.

Take the love of money, for example. When this is a tribal fault, most people from that tribe will find that they love money. They may even cheat, lie and use all sorts of cunning to acquire it. They will sacrifice people, relationships, health and all to make money. They will eat poorly, dress poorly and do everything to save and have money. A believer from such a tribe will often find that he loves money. He may even confess that he doesn't. He may even deceive himself that he doesn't, but a careful observer will sooner or later see the manifestation of this tribal fault.

So, each believer should carefully find out what is the fundamental weakness of his race or tribe and, in the name of the Lord Jesus, break loose from it. Without that kind of dealing, he may remain in the captivity of the faults of his tribe.

A believer should also find out if there were any specific activities carried out by his tribe or nation that are particularly offensive to God. For example, a people who sacrificed to idols either in the distant or recent past are an abomination to God. In some tribes people were sacrificed to Satan. Some were buried alive. Some were burnt, etc. A nation or tribe that has been hostile to the gospel and been hostile to the true servants of God, is under a curse and, to some extent, people from that nation or tribe are under a curse. This knowledge should help the believer to see what is against him, even though he himself may be without guilt. As we said before, he should see things clearly and deal with them accordingly; first of all, for his own good, secondly, for the good of his descendants and, thirdly, for the good of his tribe or nation.

PART SEVEN

Forgiving others: A key for inner healing

A lady came to our clinic. She had a problem and wanted to be prayed for. She spoke to me a little. I immediately discerned that she had another problem which was more serious than the one she was presenting to me. I asked her if she was bitter against anyone. She waited for a while and then told me, "Yes, I am bitter against my former husband. He treated me very badly and finally divorced me and made no provisions for me and the two children we had together. I hate him." Another woman said, "I am bitter against my husband because he brought another woman into our home and pays more attention to her than to me." Another said, "I am bitter against my mother-in-law. She helped to turn my husbands's heart against me." A graduate told me, "I hate one girl with my total force. She preferred another man to me and put me to public shame. Each time I think of her, anger wells up in me and I long for revenge." Another man said, "My boss stood in my way and so I was not promoted. I am waiting for the day when I shall hear of his death and then I shall celebrate." Another man said, "This government threw me out of my job and shut me up in a cell. While I was in prison, I lost everything. I am waiting for the day that it shall be toppled and may it be soon. I would like it to be a bloody take over and may whoever takes over be a ruthless destroyer who would spare no one. Then I shall be happy."

All these statements come from people who are bitter. They were probably wronged by someone and they kept the wrong in their hearts and nourished it. They bear a grudge against someone or some group of people. They have not forgiven those who wronged them. They would like the people concerned to be punished for the evil they did to them.

THE DANGERS OF AN UNFORGIVING SPIRIT

An unforgiving spirit is one of the greatest liabilities that anyone can afford to have. An unforgiving spirit will destroy its owner in two major ways: it will lead to spiritual death and it may lead to physical death in the long run.

The Bible says, *"For if you forgive men their trespasses, your heavenly Father also will forgive you; but if you do not forgive men their trespasses, neither will your heavenly Father forgive your trespasses"* (Matthew 6:14-15). *"And whenever you stand praying, forgive, if you have anything against anyone; so that your Father also who is in heaven may forgive your trespasses. But if you do not forgive, neither will your Father who is in heaven forgive your trespasses" (Mark 11:25-26). "So also my heavenly Father will do to everyone of you, if you do not forgive your brother from your heart"* (Matthew 18:35).

The Word of God is plain on the matter: those who do not forgive those who wrong them will themselves not be forgiven by the Lord. They may confess their sins to Him but, as there is someone whom they will not forgive, they will not be forgiven by the Lord. So, a person can forgive and then be forgiven or he can be unforgiving and have his sins retained against him by the Lord. If the Lord does not forgive anyone, that one is lost. This means that the one who has chosen not to forgive has also chosen to perish. Those who do not forgive are harbouring sin in their hearts and, as such, the Lord cannot hear them. Dear saint, this should make you see that forgiving those who have hurt you is not an optional affair. It is basic to spiritual life.

In this matter of forgiving those who have hurt you, it is not a matter that depends upon the fact that they have seen their wrong, repented of it and come to you for forgiveness. The forgiveness that the Bible here talks of, depends on you and not on those who have wronged you. It is the type of forgiveness that was manifested on the cross by the Lord when He prayed for His unrepentant crucifiers, saying, "Father, forgive them; for they know not what they do" (Luke 23:34). To a certain extent, they knew what they were doing. At another level, they did not know what they were doing; for the god of this world had blinded their eyes. So, the Lord did not wait for them to repent and ask for pardon. He forgave them when there was no indication that they intended to repent. All believers are called to forgive in the same spirit.

The Bible demands that forgiveness be from the heart. It is not just words. I once read the story of two people who had quarrelled. Their relationship was broken for years. None of them did anything to restore the relationship. One day, one of the two men fell sick and felt that he could die. He sent for the other man and asked that they should make peace. The other man agreed and they shook hands as a symbol that their quarrel was over. No sooner had they removed their hands from each other's grasp than the man who was sick said, "This reconciliation does not stand if I do not die." He was prepared to act out a reconciliation, meanwhile, the forgiveness that the Lord wants must be deep and thorough. It must be from the heart. Since not forgiving is a sin, the act of bearing a grudge or being unforgiving must be confessed to the Lord as a sin, and cleansing sought. Then confession might have to be made to the person against whom the sin was committed. When this sin is being confessed to man, there should be no attempt to justify it. It is not a matter of going to someone and saying to him, "You did this and that against me. You were wrong, but I forgive you." It is a matter of going to someone with a broken and contrite heart and falling before him and saying to him, "I sinned against God and against you by harbouring an unforgiving attitude towards you. It is all my fault. I am guilty. Please forgive me."

Those who are repentant of the sin of having an unforgiving heart will not justify themselves. They will not even tell the person what led to the sin. They will confess it thoroughly. The reason that they would not expose the wrong that was done against them is that they see clearly that, regardless of whatever wrong was done to them, they have no justification, whatsoever, to be unforgiving. The truly repentant do not justify their sin in any way. They do nothing to palliate the wrong that they have done. They see themselves as having sinned, even if the other party is ninety-nine percent at fault.

The repentant put things right at once. They forgive immediately, even if they do not feel like it. They will forgive and carry out acts that befit forgiveness, regardless of how they feel. They move with their wills and thus cause their emotions to follow.

When a person forgives, he releases healing power. He is the first beneficiary from the healing power that is released by his forgiving someone. While there was the barrier between him and another person, part of his being was as if imprisoned. With the act of forgiveness, life flows anew into all of his being and the wounds that were caused by his sin of not forgiving, receive a healing touch.

An unforgiving spirit may lead to physical death. When a person meets someone against whom he holds a grudge, he gets disquieted from within. His body secretes substances that are toxic and harmful to his health. His blood pressure may rise. The initial hurt that was caused by the act that led to unforgiveness deepens and the wound expands. He becomes restless and his peace is gone. Things worsen as the one whom he has not forgiven prospers. He may say many evil things against the person and wish him a lot of evil in his thoughts. The unforgiven party knows nothing about the thoughts and the words that are harboured or spoken against him, and so is unaffected by them. However, the one who is bitter fires bullets against himself with every negative thought, wish or desire. He is, finally, the sufferer in the spiritual and physical realm.

We can sum this up by saying that a person with an unforgiving heart is doing terrible harm to himself at all levels. He should repent of this sin, confess it, forsake it and carry out restitution. He will receive inner healing for himself. He will also minister inner healing to the one he has forgiven; for, by opening himself up to loving the person and being loved by him, he blesses him.

PART EIGHT

The impact of childhood on adult life

Many people are governed by things that happened to them in their childhood. Consider the following examples:

A young girl came back from school at the end of the term. She had done well. She was the first of the girls in her class. However, the first positions in the class were taken up by boys. Her father asked her why she did not do better than she did. She explained that all those who were ahead of her were boys. Her father then told her, "From this day, you should know that you are my boy." She believed him and began behaving like a boy in every way. When she got married, she took the position of the "husband" and her husband had to become the "wife". Her decisions in the home were final and those who lived in the home knew that, if she said one thing and her husband said a different thing, it was better to obey her than him, for all who obeyed him instead of her got into trouble. Sometimes, she would determine to be the woman, but her actions and everything were still masculine. She was still the little girl who was told, "You are my boy." As far as that aspect of her life was concerned, she had never grown beyond that day, even though she had matured in very many ways. She needed inner healing. She was governed by that statement from her father declaring her a boy. She had buried the statement deep down into her being without realizing it, and it had slowly but surely transformed her into a "man".

Someone said, "For years I had been vaguely conscious of the fact that it was hard for me to care deeply for people. What troubled me most about this was that, although I dearly loved my wife and my mother, there seemed to be a point beyond which I could not let them into my heart. One day, returning from Europe by boat, my wife and I were sitting in the sun and enjoying the feeling of having nothing to do. Suddenly, it occurred to me to ask God why I could not care for people as I longed to do. So I did. Almost at once my face flushed, my hands trembled, and I grew hot and angry. I was ten years old again, and vividly reliving an experience I had completely forgotten. I had asked a little girl to be my best girl - since each of the other boys had one. She had said, "No. I like Lawrence better." I felt again all the anger and the deep hurt to my pride. I recalled abruptly turning away. The next day her closest friend had offered to be my best girl. "No," I had told her, "I don't want one - ever." During the few seconds that I so intensely relived this incidence, I could almost hear my unconscious mind register this decision: "Never again will I be hurt like that, never will I care enough for any girl to let her hurt me."

A baby girl was born outside of wedlock. Her mother never really had a husband of her own. She laboured to let her have everything. She gave her everything she wanted. She never disciplined her. She was over-indulgent with her. When she grew up, she wanted everyone to praise her and pay her much attention. She was hard on all the men who came her way. She had declared in childhood that she would revenge her mother for all the hurt that she had received from men. When she got married, she wanted to possess her husband in an absolute way. Any relationship that her husband built with anyone seemed to threaten her.

A child grew up with parents who always criticized him. They found fault with everything that he did. They never congratulated him on anything that he did well. He therefore grew up to believe that he was a failure. He however did not want to appear as a failure. He therefore decided to show off and put up a superior attitude. He treated everyone with contempt. He insisted on his way in everything. He wanted always to be seen, praised and well spoken of.

As he grew up he shunned the company of anyone whom he thought was better than he. He got married but laboured to dominate his wife in everything . He rejected all her suggestions, even when he saw the reason in what she was saying. He would never listen to another. He was still the small boy who was rejected by his parents as a failure, even though he had risen to a position of responsibility in the government. He was yearning to be accepted, yearning to prove that he was not a failure. He thought more qualifications and a better job would solve the problem, but even when he was a very senior civil servant he was insecure.

Another boy was sent by his parents to live with relatives who did not love him. In fact, they treated him very badly. He felt totally rejected. He reacted to this by withdrawing into himself. Later on, he found that he could do well in school. He decided to make a name for himself in the academic world. He studied and studied. He was always frantic about his work. He became a university lecturer and started labouring to become a professor. He worked hard and continued to be so restless that he complained about everything: his wife, his job, the administration, the financial system, the promotion board, etc. Then he developed high blood pressure and this caused him to worry even more.

I was invited to speak at a Christian conference for University students in an African country. The Lord's presence was mighty in our midst. On the third day of the conference, one of the lady students asked that I should come to the dormitory where the ladies were staying and pray for one of the girls who had come for the conference but had not attended any of the meetings. I went with her and met this young lady of about twenty-one. She was beautiful in every way. I talked to her. She told me that she was afraid of everyone. I asked her to tell me about herself. She spoke briefly. Her parents had abandoned her at the age of six and gone to Great Britain to study. She was brought up by her grandmother. She felt totally unwanted by her parents. After seven years they came back with big degrees and professional qualifications. They brought her very many things. They sent her to the best school in the nation. They did all they could, but the harm caused by those seven years of abandonment was deep. She increasingly withdrew into herself and rejected all the love that was shown to her. She became very frightened and threatened by the presence of people. Her parents sent her to Britain to see a psychiatrist, but all was to no avail. By the time I saw her that day, she seemed a hopeless case.

A woman lost her husband and had to bring up her children alone. She found one of the boys especially difficult and so she rejected him. She would blame him for everything that went wrong. If something was lost, she would immediately accuse him as the guilty party. Later on, this boy accepted the idea that he was a thief. He then began to steal. He stole so much that he became a major problem until he was invaded by a power beyond that of man.

In a family of four children, all of them boys, the parents preferred the first three children who did well at school and rejected the fourth child because he did poorly. They sometimes called him " a curse from God, problem child", etc. He received no love whatsoever. Having received no love, he grew up to be a hard man who showed no mercy on anyone. He had received no love and so he could not give any. He continued in that condition and his wife, children and relatives felt the impact of the love that had been denied him.

We could go on and on to give examples that show clearly that most people are reacting as a result of what happened to them in childhood. Those who were loved and knew that they were loved found it easier to receive and to give love in adult life. Those who were denied love seemed to spend all their lives looking for love. Many who lost their mothers early in life wanted their wives to be both lover and mother! Those who were rejected seemed to spend all their lives looking for acceptance. A young man at the age of twenty-eight found that he only associated with people who thought he was wonderful. He would announce the slightest compliment that he received to everyone. He sought always to display his talents. He would associate and build a relationship, but each time, when the person showed him any of his faults, he would break the relationship and start another one. When criticized, he would feel as if his world had collapsed. When he was converted to Christ, a lot of his character changed. However, even after many years in the Lord, he was still labouring to be seen and to run away from any helpful criticism. When he went to see someone for inner healing, it was found that his problem stemmed from the fact that he was an illegitimate child and felt deeply insecure. In childhood, he used to feel horrible embarrassed when other boys talked about their fathers and asked him where his own father was. He thus felt that he was a failure. He grew up with this attitude and, therefore, desperately wanted to be accepted as he was. He also wanted to be seen as a success in order to cover up the gnawing sense of failure for being " a boy without a father."

A girl was brought up by her mother because her father had died early in life. They lived in abject poverty. As the girl grew up, things improved, but the damage had already been done. She clung to things. Her house was filled with things - useful things and useless ones. She did everything she could to make money. She was thoroughly calculative. She counted everything. She laboured to spend less and less and keep more and more. She became literally a prisoner of things. To make things worse, she deceived herself that she was generous.

A woman of forty told her counsellor, "I always walk backwards towards a mirror. I hate to look at my face in the mirror. I do not know when I last looked at it. It is ugly. I hate it." The counsellor was surprised because her face was beautiful. He asked her why she felt that way. She told him, "Someone told me when I was five years old that my face was like that of a boy and I have believed it all these thirty-five years. I believe that my face is strong and manly. Sometimes I think that I am a man in a skirt. I have waited these years to be married and no one ever came along. No one has ever loved me. No one has ever told me that I was beautiful. Sometimes I am told that my dress is beautiful or that it fits well but those are my clothes. It is not I who is beautiful. It must be true that I am a man in a gown."

The far-reaching impact of childhood on adult life demands that children be treated with care. I went to see a family who had just had their sixth child. She was also their sixth baby girl. The man was so disappointed that he did not even take the child in his arms. She might suffer deep rejection. On the other hand, a family that has had five boys may have a daughter as a sixth child. She would then be treated with so much indulgence that she might grow up to be an adult baby, always wanting attention! There is no substitute for parents receiving Christ and obeying Christ in the treatment of their children!

How can the problems of chilhood and their impact on adult life be handled? We shall look at the answer in the next chapter.

PART NINE

God's provision for the problems of childhood

Man often tries to solve the problems of childhood on his own. This is what many psychiatrists are trying to do. They may bring some relief, but for a deep and permanent solution, man must turn to a source beyond man. He must turn to God. God can solve all the problems, and His solutions go to the root of the matter. They are deep and permanent.

For the solutions of God to become applicable, man must co-operate with God. We suggest the following steps to anyone who needs God's help to be healed from problems of the impact of his childhood on his adult life.

1) You must accept that you have been greatly influenced by your childhood. Maybe you have never thought about it. Have you ever asked yourself why you react the way you do? Maybe you are stingy, proud, stubborn, fearful, difficult to please, intolerant, restless, hard on men or on women, thoughtless, hard, etc. It could even be that you want to draw close to people but always find yourself disgusting them; you want to love but find yourself hating; you want to be tender but, before you realize, you have issued a hard word, etc.

2) You should identify where your problem lies. You should ask yourself, "Why do I react this way? Why do I find it hard to accept people? Why do I find it hard to accept criticisms? Why do I try to give people a false impression of myself? Why am I always trying to receive attention and to let people think of me as successful? Why do I resent a certain type of people and draw close to another type?"

3) You should accept your problem as it is. Pretending will never help you. If you feel insecure because you were born outside of wedlock, you should accept the fact that that is where your problem lies. If you are stingy because you grew up under very poor conditions, you should accept that that is where things are wrong. If you were

unwanted by your parents because you were the wrong sex or because you came at a time when they did not want any baby, you should accept that fact. If others were preferred to you, you should admit it. You should say, "This person or that one was preferred to me and I felt hurt."

4) If you do not know where your problem lies or from where it originated, you should ask the Lord to show you. The fact is that hurts that occurred in childhood were buried inside you. They did not disappear. They only went into the subconscious part of you. Although they were buried, they remained in you and have been actively controlling you, without your knowledge. Because many of these things happened in childhood, they might have been buried for very many years; so that you do not know them. You see their impact and you accept them as your character. That is not your true character as God meant it to be. God meant you to be like the Lord Jesus. God wants to heal you; so that your character may be like that of the Lord Jesus.

Although God can heal people who ask Him in a general way to heal them, He prefers to heal people who bring specific needs to Him. That is why it is important that you know where the root cause of your problem is. The Holy Spirit is willing and able to bring to your memory all that you need to know about your past in order to be healed. He is willing to transfer events, things, etc, from the subconscious where they were buried and from where they have controlled you without your knowing, to the conscious; so that you can know them and be healed from them.

Although the Holy Spirit is willing and able to bring things from the subconscious into the conscious, He often does not do it until He is asked. You should, therefore, ask Him to bring to your conscious mind, all that is buried deep inside you that needs to be healed. I suggest that you should take some time away from people and be alone. The time that you choose should preferably be a time during which you are relaxed and free from all pressures, including the pressure of time. You may need to ask Him and wait before Him for long before He shows you things. This is often because He often waits for people to be calm before Him and to be shut off from all the distractions of their environment. You may find it necessary to ask Him to render your being calm before Him. He will do it. You should then ask Him to show you the things that are buried in you that you need to know in order to receive healing. After you have asked, wait before Him. To avoid being distracted, you can whisper silently, "I love You, Lord Jesus. I adore You. I worship You. I honour You. I extol Your Holy Name. I am waiting on You. You will show me things through Your Holy Spirit who dwells in me. Do it now, Lord. I am waiting before You...." If you are mature in waiting before the Lord, you may not need the above words. You could just wait before Him in silence. Some people find that they need to read a Psalm or sing a song of praise in order to be able to wait before Him. Whatever method you use, make sure that you wait before Him.

As you are waiting before Him, often He will bring a scene that happened in your childhood to you. You will see what happened. It may be the moment when someone told you that you were ugly or that you would never succeed. As you see the scene, thank God for it and preferably write what the Spirit of God has shown you. You should then ask Him to show you how that event in your childhood has affected you. He will make you understand. If you do not understand, you may discuss it with someone who is spiritually competent to help you.

5) Thank God that that event took place in your life. The event may be horrible. It may be the death of your mother. It may be the fact that you were born outside of wedlock. It may be the fact that your parents did not want you because they wanted a child of a sex that was different from yours, etc. Say to the Lord, "Thank You, Lord, that I was born outside of wedlock. Thank You, Lord, that I was an unwanted baby, etc." Say to the Lord, "As I thank You, I accept full well that I was born outside of wedlock or that I was re-

jected. I am a bastard; I am the rejected one. I know these things and I accept myself as such and I thank You for it all."

You may ask, "How can I thank God for things that were done outside of His will like the sin of my parents that led to my being born outside of wedlock?" There are a number of reasons why you must thank the Lord. The first reason is that the Bible says, *"Give thanks in all circumstances; for this is the will of God in Christ Jesus for you. Do not quench the Spirit"* (1 Thessalonians 5:18-19). The Bible again says, *"Always and for everything giving thanks in the name of our Lord Jesus Christ to God the Father"* (Ephesians 5:20). It again says, *"And whatever you do, in word or deed, do everything in the name of the Lord Jesus, giving thanks to God the Father through him"* (Colossians 3:17). Because the Bible commands that thanks should be given in all circumstances and for everything, those who love the Lord obey without further questions. The second reason is that, healing from the problems caused by childhood experiences is a work of the Holy Spirit. He works when He is not quenched. Those who do not thank the Lord for everything and in all circumstances quench the Holy Spirit (1 Thessalonians 5:19) and if He is quenched, He is rendered relatively less active in healing. The third reason is that, thanksgiving in everything and in all circumstances is an act of surrender to the Lord. It says, "Lord, I believe that You knew that this event would happen. You could have stopped it, but You decided not to. Although You knew that the event was not good, You allowed it to happen because You decided that You would use it to do something in me that is greater than the harm that the event has caused. Lord, You are able to produce a gem out of a tragedy. I thank You for the tragedy because of the good that You will use it to produce in me."

The person who has thanked God for that event no longer hates the event. He no longer wants to hide the event. He is no longer ashamed of the event or of the consequence of the event. He accepts the event. He accepts himself as he is, even before he is healed. All pretence is totally abandoned. This makes the next step easy and possible.

6) Open up to someone. It is not enough to see the event or events that are the cause of life's problems and to thank the Lord for them. It is necessary to share them with someone. How do you choose the one with whom to share what your problem is? I suggest the following criteria:

a) He should be someone of spiritual maturity who knows the word of God and can use it effectively.
b) He should be someone whom you trust and feel secure to share your deepest self with.
c) He should be someone who loves you enough to be able to tell you the truth about yourself without fear.
d) He should be someone who has at least once in his life opened up deeply to someone else and, therefore, will not treat what is said to him lightly.
e) He should be someone who is prepared and able to listen and not a prejudiced person who has prefabricated answers.
f) He should be someone who is prepared to stand by you until your healing is complete, without rejecting you or be coming mechanical because you are taking too much of his time.
g) He should be someone who knows how to minister in total dependence on the Holy Spirit.

When you go to someone to open up to him, you should be honest. Tell him everything. If you do not think that you can tell him everything, do not go to him at all. In inner healing, any information that is withheld may be just that which is necessary for the healing. So, let the one who is standing with you for your healing know all that is important, even if it makes you look small. To look at it in another way, you are a patient and if you tell the doctor only part of the story, you will receive only part of the remedy or the wrong treatment.

I have found people who love flattery, are superficial in relationships, have a tendency to start but not finish projects, have an unusual attraction to the opposite sex, feel inferior and pretend by acting big and superior, who know these things about themselves but would not admit that they are that way. Ministering to them is, consequently, difficult, for they are still prepared to be false.

7) Call upon the Lord. It is not enough to share your problem with someone else, good as that may be. Opening up is bringing the problem to the surface so that it can be solved, but bringing it to the surface does not impart healing. A wound that is exposed is made ready for healing, but it is not healed just because it is exposed. It must come in contact with the appropriate drug. Jesus Christ is the Healer. He must be brought in. The person needing healing should pray presenting his hurt or wound to the Lord. The person standing with him should also pray with him and pray for him. As they bring the hurt to Jesus, they should believe Him to heal. The Bible says, *"Jesus Christ is the same yesterday and today and for ever"* (Hebrews 13:8).

Faith is as important in inner healing as it is in physical healing. The Bible says, *"And without faith it is impossible to please him. For whoever would draw near to God must believe that he exists and that he rewards those who seek him"* (Hebrews 11:6). Without faith in the Lord Jesus, who alone can heal the memories and take away the things that have been buried in the subconscious for years, resulting in diverse prejudices, tendencies, hurts, barriers, openings, etc, exposing things to Him and praying over them is useless. There is no magic in talking about your problem with someone, although that might lead to and often leads to temporary relief. That is not the healing that Jesus has in mind. He heals at the deepest level, and what He does lasts. It cannot be overthrown.

8) As you receive your healing from the Lord by faith, ask Him to grant that that part of your personality that was hindered from growing, should be caused to grow rapidly, so that all of your character and personality may synchronize to the glory of God. For example, a person who was stingy because of hard childhood conditions will receive liberation and become generous. The person who put on an

attitude of superiority to cover his inferiority will throw away that mask and manifest the humility of the Lord, etc.

As in physical healing, the symptoms of the disease may disappear immediately or they may disappear gradually. However, those who bring their problem to Jesus will receive immediate healing from Him, and the signs will follow either immediately or afterwards.

As I write this, a new joy flows in my heart. I see the possibility of many of the "character diseases" of God's children being healed. Some character diseases that I saw in myself and in others will go at once or gradually as they are brought to the Lord Jesus. Jesus will indeed have His Bride without spot, blemish or wrinkle. Glory be to His name! Amen.

So do not remain a baby in some aspect of your personality. Bring all of yourself to the Lord Jesus for perfect healing. He will do it. Why not now?

PART TEN

Rejection in adult life and healing from it

Many of the problems that we have shown as having impact on a child's life and being manifested through adult life may continue to happen in adult life. The question then arises. How can a person receive healing from the hurts that come with rejection in adult life?

There are clear steps that can lead to healing. We shall present them as clearly as we can.

First of all, rejection did not need to lead to a wound or hurt. The person who has entered into a life of perpetual inner health can be rejected one hundred times in one day and not be hurt even one time. Such a person has been delivered completely from self and there is nothing of self left in him to be hurt. (All hurts are essentially wounded self-love and the one who has been completely delivered from self-love by the Lord is totally free from self and, therefore, from any hurts in the future.) We shall say something more about the life that is totally freed from hurts in the last chapters. That is the ultimate answer to the need for inner healing. Because many believers have not yet attained unto that position, we shall deal here with the situation that is not the lot of most believers.

When a person is rejected in adult life, be it a wife who is no longer wanted by her husband, or a friend who has been let down, or a businessman who has been betrayed by a partner; of the numerous situations that can cause inner hurt, the first thing is to be honest and own up to the fact that one has been rejected. No one is healed by pretending that something that has happened has not happened. Therefore, be honest and say, "I have been rejected ." It is better to be more exact and say, "I have been rejected by this person over this issue."

The rejection is a fact, and not to admit it is falsehood. However, to be rejected is not to be hurt. There are many situations under which you may be rejected and it would not mean a thing to you.

You just go about as if nothing happened. This is the experience of those who have entered into perfect inner health. The Lord Jesus was not wounded when Peter rejected Him and made a three-fold confession that he did not know Him. He was surely rejected, but He was not wounded or hurt. Other people can be rejected and not be hurt if they are rejected by people who do not mean anything to them; for a person is often most likely to be hurt by those he loves, those to whom his self-love is most displayed.

When the rejection is noticed, a person should face the facts, and ask, "Am I hurt by this rejection or not?" Again, honesty is important. To be hurt and deceive yourself that you are not hurt is self-deception. It will not lead to healing. It will lead to greater problems in the future. It is important that the believer should ask the Lord to give him the capacity to be truly honest and to know himself. If he is prone to pretending, he may pretend without knowing that he is pretending. Falsehood then becomes his way of life, so that even when he is hurt he may deceive himself that he is not.

When the hurt is acknowledged, two pathways are opened to the one who is hurt.

1). To bury the hurt or cover it and plan to react to it. Take, for example, someone is slighted and is hurt. He then says, "I know I am not wanted by this person. I will withdraw from him. I will treat him from a distance..." By this process the hurt is buried. It will affect the person's reaction to that person in the future. It will also affect the person's reaction to other people; for what has been buried becomes a cancerous cell that will grow and affect other cells. It will cripple the person in other areas; for it will make him begin to fear and distrust other people, apart from the one who hurt him. By burying the hurt, he has allowed a simple act carried out by someone to have a formative influence on his character. We have known people in places of responsibility who worked hard to frustrate a nation or tribe because one person from that nation or tribe hurt them. We have known people who became fearful and withdrawn for many years because someone made a negative comment about their look or about something they had done. The greatest harm that anyone can do to himself is to bury the hurt and then act by reaction.

2) To expose the hurt at once to the Lord and say to Him, "Lord, this thing has hurt me. I want to remain normal. Take away this hurt from me now and give me power to forgive the person who has hurt me now."

The person who decides to have the hurt dealt with by the Lord could pray as we have suggested above. If he does that, he will be freed from the hurt at once. If he is not able to deal with the situation at once (we recommend that each hurt be brought to the Lord at once, for fresh wounds heal faster than ulcers), he should withdraw to a quiet place and talk to the Lord about it.

Normally, we recommend that people deal with the Lord directly in order to avoid gossip. However, there are some people who may not have enough faith to receive healing directly from the Lord by presenting their hurt directly to Him. We encourage such people to go to the person who hurt them, if he is a believer, and say to him, " You said this thing or did that thing. Most likely you did not mean to hurt me, but I am hurt. I have come to share it with you so that you may pray for my healing." The person may apologize for what he said or did, or he may not because he feels that you needed the word that was said to you. He will, nevertheless, pray that you should be healed of the hurt. If the person who caused the hurt is not a believer, we recommend that you seek help from a mature believer who will pray with you for your healing.

It is possible to be healed of the hurt partially. Partial healing is the situation where you remember clearly what happened to you, but it does not hurt you. That is the situation with most believers. However, God has something better than that for His children. The Lord says, *"I will remember their sins and their misdeeds no more"* (Hebrews 10:17). God can forget. He is willing to give His children the capacity, both to be healed and to completely forget that the hurt ever took place.

In this way, a person can go through life without harbouring hurts. As we said about things that happened in childhood, God is able to bring to memory things that happened in the past and have been buried; so that they are done away with. Each person should follow the same procedure and let the Lord bring the things that happened to him and which have been buried under the surface, so that they can be dealt with. Things that are buried, be they in childhood or in adult life, are dangerous.

We mentioned the fact that a person should take his hurt alone to the Lord. Let us make some clarification. We are not trying to minimize the ministry of another member of the Body of Christ to the one who is hurt. We are not trying to ask believers to prove to be self-sufficient or to develop the attitude that says that everything will be settled only between the individual and the Lord. We are simply suggesting that hurts can be healed immediately by the Lord and that people do not need to carry them for long. We are merely suggesting that no sharing of a hurt should be carried out that leads to gossip or to the exposure of the faults of one person X, by another person Y to a third person Z in the absence of X; for that would be sin.

If a person is hurt and needs to share his hurt with another person but refrains from it because he is too proud to let others know that he is hurt, the Lord will not heal him until he shares his hurt with another and they pray together. The reason for this is obvious. A person is hurt when his "self" is wounded somewhere. If the self is wounded and the person wants to hide the fact that it is wounded, it means that the person wants to continue in the "self" life. The Holy Spirit will not help him to receive healing while maintaining the "self" in him intact.

In this connection, we must add that hurt and healing should not be converted into a mechanical process. It should not become something in which, when a person is hurt, he runs to the Lord to save him from the hurt. Every hurt, whatever may be its source, is permitted by the Lord. He permits it so that the rejection may contribute to the "decentralization of self"; to the putting to death of the self - life, to the deflation of the baloon of self-love. If the Lord allows the rejection with that purpose in view, then those who are going to make the most progress are not those who will immediately seek relief, but those who will act as follows:

1. Acknowledge the fact that they are rejected.
2. Acknowledge the fact that they are hurt.
3. Acknowledge the fact that it is the "self" that has been hurt and nothing else.
4. Refuse to blame, accuse or say anything against the person through whom the rejection came.
5. Thank the Lord for the rejection.
6. Repent that the "self" life is still so abundant in them that they can be hurt in that way.
7. Ask the Lord to show them that aspect of their being that needs to die to self and for which the Lord permitted the rejection, and the Lord will show them.
8. Ask the Lord to help them put that aspect of the "self" life in their person to death.
9. Ask the Lord to enable them to make the most benefit of the rejection for the formation of christian character.
10. Ask the Lord to rapidly deal with the self that is in them, so that they will soon enter into perfect inner health.
11. Ask the Lord to take away the wound or hurt as soon as His purpose for allowing it has been accomplished, so that the enemy may not use it for his godless purposes.

It becomes obvious that, from the moment a person believes in the Lord Jesus, God will allow him to be rejected. The purpose of the rejection is that "self" may be put out of the centre of life. The purpose is that the believer should abandon his own will,

plans,
ambitions,
ways,
etc,
and seek the Lord's will, plans, ambitions and ways. When a person is rejected, it is part of this
my will,
my plans,
my ambitions,
my ways,
etc,

being put aside. God will work towards that goal. If the believer sees it, he will consider rejection as a friend. He will wait before the Lord and receive from Him how to react to each experience of rejection, so that God's great purpose for him is accomplished. God will show him how to react and, as he obeys, he will react God's way and will grow in Christ-likeness, which is also selflessness. If he reacts as the Lord wants him to react, there will be no hurts caused that need healing. When hurts occur that need healing, he should realize that he did not act as he ought to have acted. He should then repent, ask for forgiveness, act as he ought to have acted, and then receive healing from the wound that was caused, not by the rejection, but by a wrong reaction to the rejection.

We recommend that you see in each rejection an opportunity to be delivered from the monster "self" and not as an occasion to be hurt! This is the way of the cross! Do not escape from it.

PART ELEVEN

Comparison and its consequences

One thing that is prevalent among fallen people is the sin of comparison. Much heart-ache, bitterness, frustration and the like are caused by this one sin. Covetousness is at the very root of the sin of comparison. Comparison manifests itself in the following ways;

1 Someone is the first in the class and you want to be the first like him.

2 Someone is tall and you are short. You compare yourself to him and find that you do not have his height. You are no longer satisfied with your height; you want his height. You covet his height and then become frustrated because you cannot add to your height.

3 Someone is promoted. You, too, want to be promoted. You covet his promotion and become dissatisfied.

4 Someone buys a big car. You have a small car. You covet his car and begin to pray that God should give you a big car. You may amass all the reasons that you can to impress upon the Lord that you need the car for His glory, but if you would be honest, you will acknowledge that you are not seeking God's glory but yours.

5 Someone has four children. You have none. You covet his children. You may even say, "I got married before him, why is it that he has four children and I have none?"

6 Someone's children are doing very well at school. Yours are not doing as well. Ever so often you shout at your children, "Do you not see how well the children of so-so-and -so are doing at school? Can you not be like them?" You are, thereby, coveting the good performances of the children of another.

7 Someone said, "Everyone is slim. I do everything to stay slim but I always get fat. I wish I were like those girls who can eat anything that they like and yet remain slim." She was coveting the size of those who could eat anything and remain slim.

8 A woman once told her husband, "Those who started work with you at the same time are all riding cars. You have gone nowhere. I am here doomed to mud eternally." The man wanted to be like the other men. He stole money in order to buy a car and landed in prison. She was coveting the cars of the other people.

9 A father told the son, "Other people marry beautiful women. All you can bring to this compound is ugliness personified." He was comparing the physical appearance of his daughter-in-law with that of other women, to her discredit.

The sin of covetousness is dangerous on its own. The Bible says, *"Take heed, and beware of all covetousness; for a man's life does not consist in the abundance of his possessions"* (Luke 12:15). *"Put to death therefore what is earthly in you: fornication, impurity, passion, evil desire, and covetousness, which is idolatry. On account of these the wrath of God is coming upon the sons of disobedience"* (Colossians 3:5-6). *"Be sure of this, that no fornicator or impure man, or one who is covetous (that is, an idolater), has any inheritance in the kingdom of Christ and of God"* (Ephesians 5:5). The Bible shows clearly that the covetous one is an idolater. He worships that which he covets. He cannot worship things and at the same time worship the Lord. The covetous are eternally lost, unless they repent and seek the Lord. No one who is truly a child of God can continue in covetousness.

The sin of covetousness leads to many wounds. First of all, the covetous are never satisfied. Since they are always comparing what they have with what the others have, they are never satisfied. They will always find someone who has more than they or who has something better than what they have. They will always find someone who is their better. They will, therefore, never know rest.

The covetous will always be striving after one thing or another. As they strive, they will know increasing worry. They may want clothes and have them. Then they want a new car and after the car they might want a house and then another thing. On and on, they will plunge into the search of things that can never satisfy. If it is money they want, they will initially want to acquire a certain sum. When that sum of money has been acquired, it will cease to satisfy. They will then set a new goal which, when attained, will still leave them empty. However, they will still set a new goal and so on. They will never know satisfaction in their lives and they will spend all their lives striving after wind.

A covetous man marries one woman and soon begins to wish he had married a different one entirely. The woman who would have satisfied him is just the one that he did not marry.

Because of comparison and covetousness, many people carry wounds that are caused by many unfulfilled desires. This could also apply, and it often applies in the Christian ministry. Many want to preach as Mr so-so-and -so. Others want to have a ministry like that of X. Others want to sing like K. Others want to write like Y. Others want the spiritual gifts of N. The result of this is people who are coveting the gifts and ministries of others. The harm to themselves is enormous; for they are restless and unfulfilled. They enter into ministries to which the Lord never called them, in an effort to be as influential as another person. They miss the Lord completely and all that they will receive for their apparent labours will be many stripes. The harm to the Lord's interest is overwhelming, for comparison leads to jealousy, strife and division. It leads to people lording it over the people of God.

GOD'S ANSWER TO THE SIN OF COVETOUSNESS

The root cause of covetousness is self-rejection. The answer is self-acceptance. You are a unique individual. You do not need what another person has to be your best. You do not need the car, house, diploma, height, size, etc, that another person has in order to be the best that God made you for and wants you to be.

Look carefully at the things that the people you wish to be like have. Ask yourself if you would be happier if you had them. Ask yourself if those people are happy with those things. Are they not looking for something else to make them happy?

The enemy, Satan, has worked in the hearts of people, such that all their values are misplaced. The Lord said that a man's life did not consist in the abundance of his possessions. No one knows true peace as a result of

his possessions,
position or
power.

No one knows true joy as a result of any material or intellectual acquisition. The Lord Jesus demonstrated by His life where the source of joy is. He demonstrated where the source of fulfilment lay. He said,

"Blessed are the poor in spirit, for theirs is the kingdom of heaven.
Blessed are those who mourn, for they shall be comforted.
Blessed are the meek, for they shall inherit the earth.
Blessed are those who hunger and thirst for righteousness, for they shall be satisfied.
Blessed are the merciful, for they shall obtain mercy.
Blessed are the pure in heart, for they shall see God.
Blessed are the peacemakers, for they shall be called sons of God.
Blessed are those who are persecuted for righteousness' sake, for

theirs is the kingdom of heaven.
Blessed are you when men revile you and persecute you and utter all kinds of evil against you falsely on my account. Rejoice and be glad, for your reward is great in heaven, for so men persecuted the prophets who were before you" (Matthew 5:3-12).
He did not say,
"Blessed are you when you are the first in your class.
Blessed are you when you are the most beautiful girl or the most handsome boy.
Blessed are you when you are promoted at your job.
Blessed are you when you have a big car.
Blessed are you when you are married to the most beautiful wife in the world.
Blessed are you when you have four children: two boys and two girls.
Blessed are you when your children are the first in their classes.
Blessed are you who eat large quantities and stay slim.
Blessed are you when you, like your mate, own a car so that things are easy for your wife.
Blessed are you when your son marries a beautiful girl.
Blessed are you when your bank account grows.
Blessed are you when you are the world's most sought-after evangelist, pastor, teacher, author, etc.
Blessed are you when you have the largest following.
Etc."

There is only one way to be truly fulfilled, and that one way is the way of absolute surrender to the Lord Jesus, with a determination to be in the world as He was in it. This surrender will cause the surrendered person to obey the Word of God, which says, "Seek the things that are above, where Christ is, seated at the right hand of God. Set your minds on things that are above, not on things that are on earth" (Colossians 3:1-2). This is one of the major keys to inner healing. This is how to deal with comparison, covetousness, and like passions. Before you start to compare yourself with someone and before you start to desire something, ask yourself the question, "Is this thing of above, where Christ is seated at the right hand of God?" If the thing is of above and you seek it, you will be blessed. Put all of yourself into seeking it. The more you seek it, the more your personality will become integrated and the more peace you will know. All other things are not worth seeking. They are useless. Make sure that you set your mind on the things that are above and not on the things that are of the world. Setting the mind is a definite effort, a definite act, a continuous act in one direction. Seeking means that the entire personality is plunged after one thing and all is put into it. In order to help anyone in need, we shall make two lists, one of things that are of above (heavenly) and the other of things that are below (earthly).

Heavenly things	Earthly things
1 Holiness	1 Happiness
2 Purity	2 Excitement
3 Goodness	3 Pleasure
4 Kindness	4 Money
5 Long suffering	5 Property
6 Peace with God	6 Comfort
7 Patience	7 Ease
8 Love of God	8 Honour from men
9 Love of man	9 Promotions from man
10 Winning people to Christ	10 Celebrity
11 Building people in Christ	11 Influence over men
12 Close walk with Jesus	12 Admiration by others
13 The Power of the Holy Spirit	13 Acceptance by man
14 Intimate knowledge of the Lord	14 Worldly knowledge
15 A knowledge of God's word	15 Good looks
16 Obedience of God's word	16 Praise from people
17 Friendship with God, etc	17 Etc.

If you seek heavenly things, you will be healed inwardly. If you seek earthly things, you will receive many wounds in the process. If you set your mind on heavenly things, you will increasingly become like Jesus, and He is perfectly whole. If you set your mind on earthly things, you will increasingly become like Satan who is the god of this world, and you will increasingly know hurts, frustrations and disappointments. If you want heavenly things and earthly things, you are divided at heart. You will not know inner healing. You will not know inner health.

The Lord Jesus said, *"No one can serve two masters, for either he will hate the one and love the other or he will be devoted to the one and despise the other. You cannot serve God and mammon"* (Matthew 6:24). You cannot have the praise of God and the praise of men. You cannot seek the things of heaven and the things of the world. You must choose.Those who will know deep inner healing and know continuous inner health will read the following scripture and meditate on it and apply it in their lives. *"There is great gain in godliness with contentment; for we brought nothing into the world, and it is certain that we cannot take anything out of the world; but if we have food and clothing, with these we shall be content. But those who desire to be rich fall into temptation, into a snare, into many senseless and hurtful desires that plunge men into ruin and destruction. For the love of money is the root of all evils; it is through this craving that some have wandered away from the faith and pierced their hearts with many pangs"* (1 Timothy 6:6-10).

The Bible says that there is great gain in godliness with contentment. It does not say "gain is godliness." In fact, those who seek material gain will never know contentment. They will know worry when they have no material wealth. They will know worry when they have some material wealth and they will know much worry as their material wealth increases. You brought nothing into the world. You will go back as you came - naked. You will not take

money,
diplomas,
position before men,
honour from men, etc,

with you.

You will not even take your wife, children, etc, with you!

All need food and clothing, and God has promised to provide these. The Lord Jesus said, *"Therefore do not be anxious, saying, 'What shall we eat?' or 'What shall we drink?' or 'What shall we wear?' For the Gentiles seek all these things; and your heavenly Father knows that you need them all. But seek first his kingdom and his righteousness, and all these things shall be yours as well"* (Matthew 6:31-33).

When people have food and clothing, the Bible says that they are to be content. Anyone who has food and clothing today and is anxious is an idolater. He worships that which causes him to be anxious. He worships that thing whose absence causes him to be anxious. Those who have food and clothing today are to be fully satisfied and to pray to the Lord to supply the food and clothing that they need for tomorrow when tomorrow comes. God will surely supply their need when tomorrow comes. The Bible says, *"Rejoice in the Lord always; again I say, Rejoice. Let all men know your forbearance. The Lord is at hand. Have no anxiety about anything, but in everything by prayer and supplication with thanksgiving let your requests be made known unto God. And the peace of God, which passes all understanding, will keep your hearts and your minds in Christ Jesus"* (Philippians 4:4-7).

The Lord will supply all the needs of His children who rejoice in Him always. He will supply the needs of those who are anxious about nothing but who in everything by prayer and supplication with thanksgiving make their needs known to Him. The Lord has nowhere promised to supply the luxurious desires of the greedy and covetous. Anyone who asks God to supply the things that will make him compare favourably with another person is tempting God. Those who desire to be rich

fall into temptation,
into a snare,
    into senseless desires,
    into hurtful desires

that plunge them into ruin - spiritual ruin, ruin to inner health and ruin to physical health. No one can desire to be rich and be healed of his inner hurts, without repenting and casting away that wrong desire. If you desire to be materially rich, you are doomed to remain sick inwardly. Your desire may materialize or it may not, but the fact that you desire to be rich will cause you to be sick inwardly. If the riches do not come, you will have the disease called "frustration." If the riches come, they will bring you other diseases, including the one called "restlessness."

It is not only the desire to be rich that will destroy inner health. There are many other desires that will work in the same direction. These include:

the desire to be beautiful,
the desire to be loved,
the desire to be accepted by man,
the desire to be praised,
the desire to be preferred,
the desire to be considered a success,
the desire to control and lead others,
etc.

Wherever these desires abide, they will lead the person away from the true inner health; for they will lead the person away from the Lord of health. The world has a concept of greatness which is violently opposed to that of Jesus. He said, *"You know that those who are supposed to rule over the Gentiles lord it over them, and their great men exercise authority over them. But it shall not be so among you; but whoever would be great among you must be your servant, and whoever would be first among you must be slave of all. For the Son of man also came not to be served but to serve, and to give his life as a ransom for many"* (Mark 10:42-45).

If you accept yourself as the unique person that God has made you to be, and know that what you have is enough, if you get your heart cleansed of the sin of covetousness and the tendency to compare, you will know inner healing.

There is a very real reason why you should accept yourself. The reason is that the Lord has accepted you as you are. He has indeed accepted you as you are. He has accepted you without regard to your physical looks,

financial position,
educational attainment,
etc.

Because He has accepted you as you are, you should accept yourself and be at peace. Others may not accept you, but does that matter? The God of heaven has accepted you! What is the use of the acceptance of another person? Someone may say you are not beautiful or handsome, but listen to what the Bible says about you, *"For thou didst form my inward parts, thou didst knit me together in my mother's womb. I praise thee, for I am fearfully and wonderfully made. Wonderful are thy works! Thou knowest me right well; my frame was not hidden from thee, when I was being made in secret, intricately wrought in the depth of the earth"* (Psalm 139:13-15).

There is another thought to it. Physical beauty is vain. It soon passes away. Where are the beauty queens of twenty years ago? Is it not foolish to concentrate on that which is passing away?

What of money? What is its lasting value? Where are the rich men of the past century? When they died, what became of their wealth? Are they enjoying it today?

What of fame and honour? Where are the great politicians of fifty years ago? Where are the Churchills,

Gandhis,
Nkrumahs,
etc?

Are they still bathing in popularity today? Where are they? Will you not turn wholly to the Lord and seek the contentment that He offers?

That is the way to inner healing!
That is the way to inner health!!

This is rooted in the fact that you are the best person on Planet Earth to accomplish the purpose that God created you for. You, with all that you are of strengths and weaknesses, are the very best for that purpose. The President of the greatest nation in the world will be a poor replacement of you for the task for which the Lord created you. The richest man in the world, the most educated one, the most handsome one, the most sought-after one, etc, will all be at the best, second class as far as suitability for the task for which God created you and for which He wants you, are concerned. How then can you want to be someone who is not as suitable as you are for your God-given task? You, cry out! "I am God's number one person for the purpose for which He created me. I am His. I am His very best for it. I would not want to be another person, because the best other person in the world is not as good as I am for the task for which God created me and wants me to be. If I had what he had, and became like him, I would immediately move from being the very best, into being less than the very best." With that knowledge, you should immediately see the end of the sin of comparison. You should fully accept yourself. You should immediately be delivered from inferiority complexes. You should immediately be delivered from superiority complexes, from pride, arrogance, etc. You should rededicate yourself to the Lord and say to Him, "Lord, here I am. I realize that I am the best person for the purpose for which You made me. I yield myself unconditionally to You. I realize that Your plan for my life is better than anyone that I or any other being in all creation can ever work out. I accept Your will for my life. I accept the fact that You accept me. I do not care about the acceptance of anyone else. Your acceptance is enough. Your acceptance is my joy. I will live for You in every way from now on and for ever. Glory be to Your Holy name." Amen.

PART TWELVE

Inner health in perpetuity

We have seen a bit of how to deal with hurts and disappointments. This is inner healing. Inner healing is good, but there is something better, and that is inner health.

God wants His children to be healed, but He wants even more that His children should enjoy perpetual inner health.

If you will look carefully, all that has to do with inner healing has to do with "self". When a person is hurt it is really because the self in him has been touched.

Take, for example, the fact that a person is hurt because another person was preferred for promotion. The hurt comes because his "self" that wants to be exalted has not been given an opportunity for this to happen. His "ego" has been wounded. He may refuse to see this, but that is the root of most of his problems. When a person labours to be first, is it not because he wants to say, "I did this"? Is it not because he wants to be praised? When another person wants to receive the same honour but is not able to be the first and is the second, the fifth or the last and, therefore, is frustrated and disappointed, is the disappointment not principally because the "self, the "ego", the "I" is not exalted?

Why do people labour and strive to buy expensive cars, clothes, chairs, etc? Why do they especially want to buy chairs that are imported from Europe? Why do they want "deluxe" chairs that are made locally? Why do they spend large sums of money on chairs that would serve the same function (providing something to sit on) that very simple chairs would perform? Is it not to show off? Is it not to want to be praised, noticed, accepted?Why do people invest the sums of money they do on their bodies and clothes? Why do people buy expensive clothes and spend large sums of money on changing fashion? Is it not all the desire to be seen, noticed, praised, and appreciated?

When a person is told how bad or how foolish he is and he withdraws and mourns over it, is it not because the "self" has been wounded?

When people complain, "I wore a new dress and he said nothing about it." "He prefers someone else." "He does not love me as he loves the other one." "They have a deep freezer and we do not have one." "They earn a bigger salary than us." "We started working together and now he is already a director and I am nothing." Etc. Are they not just saying that the "self", the "I", the "ego" has not been allowed to have what it wants?

When people speak evil of others, criticize them, distort what they say and paint them as black as possible, is it not to defend the self in one way or the other? Is it not a reaction out of fear that the other person may receive some honour that should come to them? Is it not self that causes people to try to destroy each other? Is it not the selfish spirit of competition that is at the root of all the restlessness of today? When people go to marriage counsellors and complain bitterly about their mates, is it not a manifestation of their "self" that has been hurt in one way or the other? What is the root cause of broken friendships, broken engagements, and broken marriages? Is it not that one person wanted something his own way and the other party wanted things her own way and the two ways were different and each clung to his way and there was a clash? Do the parties not say, "I wanted her to be like this and to do things this way and to reason that way. She is not like I wanted her to be. She does not do things the way I want and she does not reason as I do. She does not treat my children the way I want. She does not treat my relatives the way I want. She is not as slim as I want. She does not cook my type of food my way," etc. Or "He does not treat me with respect. He does not respect me. He does not seek my opinion. He does not dress the way I like. He is not at home when I need him. He sleeps when I want to talk to him. He does not enjoy my company, etc."

Do you realize how frequent the pronouns, "I", "My", "Me" occur in these sentences? Do you see the implication? I think they are clear; almost all broken relationships are due to the sin of self-centredness. Almost all problems in the domain of inner healing are due to wounded selves.

Love is strong and blind; self-love is very strong and very blind.

Many people do not realize that all their problems or most of their problems stem from self-love. They give all the other reasons. They blame everyone else. They want to change everyone else or they want everyone else to change. They do not see that they are at the root of the problems and that if they changed, things would begin to be different.

Because most problems of inner healing are associated with self in one way or the other,

be it self-love,
self-display,
self-esteem,
self-protection,
self-pity,
self-justification,
etc,

the only way to have inner health is to deal very radically and very permanently with the self. All other treatments may lead to temporary healing, but permanent healing must wait for "self" to be dealt with permanently. The one who has his "self" dealt with permanently has entered into inner health.

Such a one will not say anything to defend himself. He has nothing of himself or of self to defend. Because he has nothing of himself or of self to defend, he will not be hurt or wounded by what anyone says about him or about what he has done. If he is congratulated, he will not be elated by it. If he is blamed, he will not be discouraged or feel rejected. If he is promoted, he will take it gladly. If he is demoted, he will take it with thanksgiving. If people accept what he says, he is at home with them. If they reject what he says, he is yet at home with them. He is totally unmoved by the opinion of men. He is moved only by what God thinks. He does not labour to impress anyone. He works to satisfy the Lord. If the whole world knows about him, that does not exalt him. If no one knows about him, he is not disturbed. If people give him credit for what he has done, he is not moved by the credit. If people give the credit for what he has done to others, he is not moved. If he is corrected, he receives the correction gladly. If he is loved, he is grateful. If he is not loved, he does not seek to be loved. He does nothing to draw attention to himself. If he has failed, he exposes his failure and turns away from it. He speaks the truth and only the truth. He withholds nothing that ought to be said for fear of the consequence of speaking. He says nothing that ought not to be said, regardless of what he might gain by saying it. He rejoices with those who are honoured in preference to him and does not want to change positions with them; since he knows that he is in God's will and in God's standing. He is at rest. He is at peace. He has inner health and there is nothing that can take away his health.

The Lord Jesus was like that. He possessed perfect inner health. He never defended Himself. He never advertised Himself. He always thought about others. He did not hold Himself back. He gave Himself away.

Jesus indeed possessed inner health. He did love people. He loved those who did not love Him. He blessed those who cursed Him. He forgave His enemies without waiting for them to ask for forgiveness. He bore no hurts. A friend betrayed Him; yet He was not bitter. He knew the intention of His betrayer three years before; yet He loved him, made him the treasurer of the group, and offered him a special place of honour at the last supper.

HOW CAN A PERSON RECEIVE INNER HEALTH?

The way to inner health is the way of death to self. It is the way of the cross. The Lord Jesus denied Himself, took up His cross and died on it. He invited all who are His in the following terms, *"So therefore, whoever of you does not renounce all that he has cannot be my disciple"* (Luke 14:33). *"If any man would come after me, let him deny himself and take up his cross daily and follow me"* (Luke 9:23).So, there must be the denial of self. There must come a day in the life of the believer who would know perpetual inner health when he says to the Lord, "Today, I commit myself to a life of self-denial. I sentence to death on the cross all that demands that the "self" in me should live and manifest itself. Lord, I do this fully knowing that it works, because You took the "self" in me to the cross and crucified it there when You died in my place and I died in You." From that day, that believer is to use his mind to co-operate with the Holy Spirit to ensure that the "self" remains dead. He should renounce his rights and privileges to all that the world offers in things and positions, fully determined that he will respond to every situation as he knows Jesus would have responded. He should decide that:

1 He will never do anything to advertise himself or draw attention to himself. He should repent of any failure in this and seek cleansing from the blood.

2 He will determine not to acquire anything that he does not absolutely need. He should get rid of all items of ease and luxury. He should reshape his life style to fit that of the Lord as shown in the pages of the gospel.

3 He will decide never to defend himself or to justify himself, regardless of whether what is said about him is true or not. He has ceased to bother about the opinion of men. He bothers about what God thinks and labours to please Him in every way.

4 He will commit himself to love everyone, regardless of what the person deserves. He will love his friends and his enemies. He will love those who admire him and those who despise him, regardless of their reason for despising him.

5 He will set his heart on the things above and let those things model him. He should covet nothing.

6 He will act by conviction and not by reaction. If he has decided on a certain course of action, he must pursue that course and not be moved from it by the action or reaction of people. He first decided on that course by conviction. He dare not change as a reaction to what people have said or done. If, for example, he has decided to act with generosity towards someone, he should not change and withhold the act of generosity because the person was not grateful. If he decided to help someone in need, he must go ahead and help the person, regardless of what the person has said and done against him. If he knows that something is wrong and needs to be condemned, he must, nevertheless, condemn it, regardless of who will be affected by the denouncing of that thing. He will be warm to those who are warm towards him and he will be warm to those who are cold towards him. He will love people when they love him and he will love them when they hate him. He will speak well of those who speak well of him. He will speak well of those who say nothing about him and he will speak well of those who speak evil of him.

7 He will commit himself completely to the will of God. He will seek the will of God and he will delight in doing the will of God. Thus lost in the will of God, he will see the world and all that is in it through the eyes of the Lord Jesus and, as he becomes increasingly like Jesus, his joy will be complete and his health faultless.

8 By experiencing inner health in full measure, he will be a competent minister of inner healing.

Amen.

Imprimé en France par CPI
en septembre 2019

Dépôt légal : septembre 2019
N° d'impression : 154142